STEP RIGHT UP

By *Brooks McNamara*

STEP RIGHT UP
THE AMERICAN PLAYHOUSE IN THE EIGHTEENTH CENTURY
THEATRES, SPACES, ENVIRONMENTS
(with *Richard Schechner*
and Jerry Rojo)

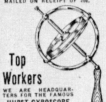
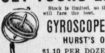

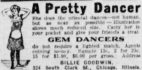

PIPES FOR PITCHMEN
By GASOLINE BILL BAKER

FORGET

By Charles I. Tryon, the Sagebrush Poet

High doodle doodle, I squandered my boodle,
My bank-roll's a thing of the past,
And with a cracked noodle, without any boodle,
How long can a damfool last?
I once lived in clover but that day is over,
And I have naught but regret;
I'll mend up my noodle and get some more boodle
And try like a man to forget.

ANENT THE ANSELME MONUMENT FUND

Just at the time when the money contributed
for the stone to be placed over Doc Anselme's
grave in St. Louis was being taken up for that
purpose Doc Hope gave us the information that
the Anselme jewels, amounting easily to $500
in value, were pledged in an Indiana town for
the sum of little more than a hundred dollars.
Doc Hope at the time suggested that if real
charity was the motive the substantial act was
to redeem the gems, for a manifold purpose.
First, to allow Mrs. Anselme to get something
like value for them, and in that way set her
on her feet and get a stone as well.
The matter was placed before all who contributed, and they were heartily in favor of
the movement. This has been the cause of the
delay.
Now it remains that we raise the difference
between $50 and $115, the required amount to
raise the jewels.
These who have contributed to the cause are:

Ed Seyler $8.00
Harry Daley 5.00
Frank Cheed 10.00
Doc and Dinah Ward 2.50
Capt. Smith 10.00
Burt Spencer 10.00
Henry Hughes 5.00
Syd Reid 1.00

John Shaud 1.00
Doc Madden 1.00
                                    _____
Total $59.50

Make the contributions payable to The Billboard Pub. Co., and put your shoulder to the
wheel and push. It is one of the most deserv-
ing causes which has yet been put forth.

Sammy Lewis, the English Duke, was seen in
New York with a rattler ducket a yard long,
heading for the depot for parts unknown. He's
still working supers.

Charlie Haskel and Misons are working in
Pennsylvania with notions. They always get
the oday no matter where they work.

Bob Lee, George Hughes, George Knobbs and
a few other old-timers were seen heading for
the Smoky City. Yes, they're all going to
frame big store shows—maybe in opposition to
some of the big department stores.

Kid Dodgin is raking in the shekels around
Williamsport passing out gyroscopes. The kid
is some talker.

Hagerstown and Frederick, Md., are good
spots to overlook. They have been first-class
bloomers for the boys. It is whispered that
Rosenberg was the only one to get any long
green there.

Chambersburg, Pa., is a good Saturday burg
—a sawbuck and worth it.

J. E. Hewitt was seen in Berk Bros. piling up
a line of stock. No, he said he wasn't going
to open a store. Just taking a little flyer into
the uncharted wilds. Jim looks healthy, prosperous and may be wealthy.

Thos. H. Haggerty, the old-time stick worker, has gone into opposition to Henry Ford. He
sells speed-'em-ups, and some good ones, too.

A few of the boys who worked at the Ithaca
Fair and afterwards blew into Rochester ar-
in arm, on the same rattler: Gummy-ga-hoo
Shalgo, Smithy, suspenders; Wilson, needle
threader worker (no relation to Wilson of hair

tonic fame); Garrison gummy-ga-hoo. They must
have gotten enough money, for they all seemed
like good fellows.

Phil Unger is cleaning up in the city of
baked beans and tea parties.

Ray Weber, the old-time manager of Kelly's
emporium is back at Twenty-third street, New
York City. Ray has been like a camel for a
week. Keep up the record the same as the
boss, Ray. Yep, Jim's off Green River.

At last our old friend, Cooley, has a B. R.
He was last seen working on upper Broadway
with tops.

The Irish Fair at Madison Square Garden, in
the big burg was Irish for fair, with the Ger-
mans mixed in. Schlitz and Green River flowed
merely to prove neutrality. At that some of
the boys got money, especially Meyer Bros.
Cooley was there and blew his joint the first
night.

Reports on the Grand Palace doings later. Fred
Nevins and his bunch were there—nuf ced.

M. A. Fingold was seen in the coal fields
working shivs. How would you like them all
like Shamokin Pa. M. A.? That's the way to
get 'em.

Jim Kelley donated a lot of stock and his
big window to help the Irish fund during its
run. We always knew that Jim was of a
philanthropic turn of mind.

Doc Burger and Fay Abbott, of the Rockner
Med. Show were seen in and out of the cos-
tumers of the loop of Chicago recently, and it
looked as if they were taking a long shot at
the spring preparedness. Fay told Doc he was

JIM FERDON'S HOME IN LOS ANGELES

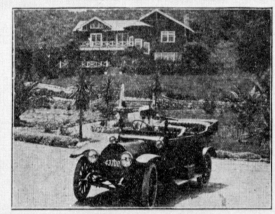

Herewith is shown the Los Angeles palace of Doc Jim Ferdon, the silver-crowned king of the med. game.
In the foreground is Jim's daughter, in the family car.

a wonderful worker and Doc told Fay she was
a wonderful entertainer. Mebbe Doc's anxious
to go on the road anyhow. More power to 'em.

Pipe this! "Told Rotarians About Rattlers,"
box-car type, and then a long tale about how
Robt. E. Lee and Charley Lee told them the
haunts and wants of the rattlers. There'll be
no limit to those boys now. Bob says the days
of centuries are still with us.

Kloe, an old-timer, whom many will remember,
has settled down in Wilkes-Barre, where he has
become famous as the paper king. He always
carries a supply of Billyboys. Give him the OO
when you jump there—and as a fixer and with
the info he's strong as horseradish.

A big mouth usually goes with a big head—
and both are hollow.

This is the stuff that pays: W. H. Moore and
Cement Reel both worked cement at the Lan-
caster Fair in perfect harmony. And it might
be added they did fine. If others of the fraternity would follow their example they would
profit as Reel and H. W. did. And H. W. and
Reel are no springers in the game.

One thing about Old Bill Stumps he doesn't
mind competition; in fact, he likes it. Bill and
Doc Livermore are still good friends and split
time at a recent Ohio Fair.

"Sister Mae—Why don't you write? I know
you are together. Mama expects some ex-
planation of your actions and I can't make any.
—Sister Marjorie."

Mrs. Doc Snyder was seen working at Forty-
seventh and Ashland in Chicago, and said business was so rotten she was willing to vote for
anybody.

Hiram Engle says that the Dutch and the
campaigners are alike—"half the lies they tell
about each other ain't so." Hiram says he thought
the White Rat stuff was bad enough, but between the two of them he's willing to pull the
covers over his head and let the country go to
the bow-wows, because he wouldn't be able to
step it anyhow if it's half as bad as they say
it is.

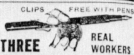
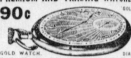

STEP RIGHT UP

Brooks McNamara

DOUBLEDAY & COMPANY, INC.
Garden City, New York
1976

Excerpt from *Him* by E. E. Cummings. Reprinted by permission of Nancy T. Andrews, courtesy of Irving Fox.

Letters on pages 200–201 from *The Youth of James Whitcomb Riley* by Marcus Dickey, copyright 1919 by The Bobbs-Merrill Company, Inc., R. 1947, reprinted by permission of the publisher.

Excerpt from *Main Street* by Sinclair Lewis. Reprinted by permission of Harcourt, Brace Jovanovich, Inc. and Jonathan Cape, Ltd.

Library of Congress Cataloging in Publication Data

McNamara, Brooks.
    Step right up.

    Bibliography: p. 215
    1. Medicine shows—History.   I.   Title.
GV1803.M32   791.1
ISBN 0-385-02959-4
Library of Congress Catalog Card Number 73–20522

To Dean Trevor

CONTENTS

ILLUSTRATIONS

PREFACE

When I was a child my grandmother often told me stories about the medicine show companies that came to the tiny town of Brimfield, Illinois, each summer during the eighties and nineties. Because they were the only traveling shows to appear in Brimfield for months and sometimes even years at a time, she recalled their visits as very special events in the life of the town. To her, even half a century later, the medicine shows were still charged with much the same air of mystery and excitement that they had possessed in her girlhood. A few years ago I decided to find out something about the shows that had interested her. The name of one remedy mentioned by my grandmother—Kickapoo Indian Sagwa—stuck in my mind, perhaps because of Al Capp's famous comic strip libation, Kickapoo Joy Juice. I discovered that the makers of Sagwa, the Kickapoo Indian Medicine Company, had indeed sent traveling shows into central Illinois at the turn of the century. But I also found that relatively little had been written about the Kickapoo shows or, for that matter, about any medicine shows.

Aside from a biography or two and a few novels, there has never been a book about the medicine show. In the twenties and thirties a number of articles by old showmen and medicine show enthusiasts found their way into print. But most were the products of casual journalism, and although they often make lively reading, the majority are impressionistic and unreliable. The number of accounts that earnestly attempted to separate fact from fiction was, I found, relatively small. Several works on quackery and patent medicine history contain good brief studies of the shows, and there are a few recent articles that deal seriously with some aspect of the history of the medicine show. But by and large, like most forms of American folk and popular entertainment, the medicine show has been neglected by scholars and writers.

As I collected more material and talked with former showmen it became apparent to me that, in spite of this neglect, the medicine show had once been amazingly widespread and influential, especially in rural areas, and that it was a unique and complicated theatrical form, a wedding of the ancient European mountebank's show and nineteenth-century American popular entertainments. Like all popular theatrical forms, however, it presented difficult research problems. For three-quarters of a century medicine show companies appeared, merged, and disappeared with frightening rapidity; showmen changed their own identities and those of their shows whenever it was convenient or necessary; the names of successful medicine show remedies were stolen or closely imitated by competitors almost as a matter of course; and systematic records were virtually nonexistent. Even the language of the medicine show is a puzzle all its own, one which I have attempted to solve to some degree in the glossary at the end of this book. Added to the confusion is the fact that in later years the medicine showman began to assume the stature of an American folk hero (or perhaps, more accurately, anti-hero), and it has become increasingly hard to distinguish the history of the medicine show from the myths that gradually grew up around it.

In spite of such difficulties, *Step Right Up* is, I hope, written with reasonable regard for accuracy about the evolution and eventual decline of the medicine show. I have tried to weed out the obvious tall tales or to label them as such, and to base my statements only on material that I was able to cross-check through several different sources. With the help of scholars, librarians, and former medicine show lecturers and performers, it has been possible to gather together, in addition to the usual research materials, such diverse items as patent medicine labels, medicine showbills, trade cards, tape recordings of songs and medicine pitches, and other artifacts. I was once even offered the loan of a pair of pitchman's gasoline torches and a patent medicine wagon.

Three of my benefactors deserve special thanks. Anna Mae

Noell, a veteran performer, has spent countless hours writing me descriptions of medicine show life and operations and setting down on paper her versions of traditional medicine show sketches, several of which appear here as appendixes. William Helfand generously opened his extraordinary private collection of pharmacy and patent medicine materials to me. From his collection came an early twentieth-century medicine showman's scrapbook which was to be one of my most important sources. Finally, I am everlastingly indebted to Professor James Harvey Young of Emory University. His excellent books and articles on patent medicine history and the history of quackery have been indispensable to me, and his generosity in supplying me with sources, notes, and encouragement for my project has been boundless.

For suggestions, help, or research materials I am also grateful to Professor David L. Cowen of Rutgers University; Susan Poston of the Hagley Museum, Wilmington, Delaware; Harry J. McLaughlin of the *Sunday Patriot News,* York, Pennsylvania; Helen Virden of the National Society for the Preservation of Tent, Folk and Repertoire Theatre; Helen Willard and Jeanne Newlin of the Harvard Theatre Collection; Mary Anne Jensen of the Princeton Theatre Collection; Louis Rachow of the Walter Hampden Memorial Library of the Players' Club; Paul Myers of the Theatre Collection, New York Public Library; Professor David Schaal of the University of Iowa; Professor Arrell M. Gibson of the University of Oklahoma; Professor Keith Clark of Central Oregon Community College; and Robert Gamble, Dan Martin, Joseph L. Barr, and Victoria Nes Kirby.

A number of former medicine show lecturers and performers and others connected with the outdoor amusement industry have generously given me interviews, written me letters, or discussed aspects of this book with me. For their help to me I am obligated to Flo St. John, Bill Smith, Bill Ruesskamp, Mr. and Mrs. Bob Styer, Bobby Snyder, Mr. and Mrs. Milton Bartok, the Mighty Atom, Walter Heeney of *Amusement Business,* and Bill Sachs, for many years the writer of "Pipes for Pitchmen," the medicine showman's column in *The Billboard.*

In addition to the libraries and museums already mentioned, additional research materials came from the Picture Collection and the Division of Genealogy and Local History of the New York Public Library, the Library of the New York Academy of Medicine, the National Library of Medicine, the Folger Shakespeare Library, the New-York Historical Society, the Museum of the City of New York, the Knox College Library, the New York University Library, the Columbia University Library, the Peoria Historical Society, the New Haven Colony Historical Society, the Umatilla County Library, the Chicago Historical Society, the University of Oklahoma Library, the Brown University Library, the Library of Congress, the Oregon Historical Society, the Newberry Library, and the Fogg Art Museum. I am grateful to the librarians and archivists in these institutions for their aid and to New York University for grants that helped to make my research possible. Some material from Chapters 5, 6, and 7 appeared in *Educational Theatre Journal*, December 1971, under the title, "The Indian Medicine Show," and a portion of Chapter 9 was printed in *Theatre Quarterly*, May–July 1974. Portions of Chapter 8 appeared in *American West Magazine*, March 1975; and of Chapter 2 in *TWA Ambassador*, October 1975. This material is reprinted here with the permission of the publishers. Four medicine show sketches ("Numbers," "Photograph Gallery," "Pete in the Well," and "Over the River, Charlie") are copyright 1974 by Anna Mae Noell and appear here with her permission.

My very special thanks go to my editors, Diane Cleaver and Sally Arteseros for their help and kindness, and to members of my family for their continuing interest in this project. It sometimes seems to me that most of my relatives have been involved with this book in one way or another. It began with the stories told by my grandmother, Elizabeth Barry; my parents, Margaret and Elmer McNamara, sent me information on the career of Jim Lighthall; and my uncle, the late Dean Trevor, to whom this book is dedicated, gave me recollections of Dakota medicine shows. My mother-in-law, Nan Jansen, patiently typed the manuscript of *Step Right Up* and quietly corrected my spelling errors. Just for the record I would like her to know that her daughter Nan provided the kindness and understanding that ultimately made this book a reality.

Brooks McNamara
NEW YORK UNIVERSITY

Step right up—here you are! You may not have cinderella but if you haven't it's a cinch you've got something else and no matter what it is this little box will save your life one dose alone irrevocably guaranteed to instantaneously eliminate permanently prevent and otherwise completely cure toothache sleeplessness clubfeet mumps stuttering varicoseveins youthful errors tonsilitis rheumatism lockjaw pyorrhea stomachache hernia tuberculosis nervous debility impotence halitosis and falling down stairs or your money back.

e. e. cummings, *Him*

STEP RIGHT UP

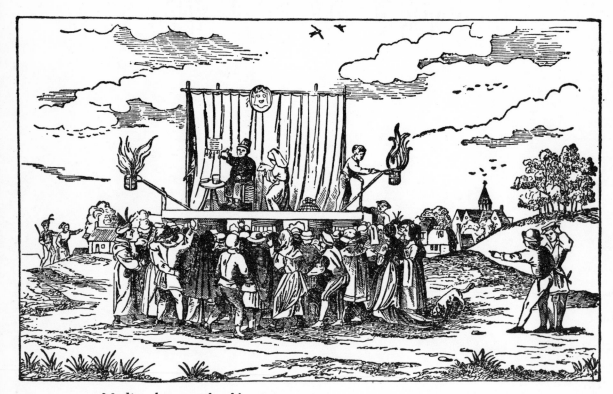

Medieval mountebank's stage.

1

STEP RIGHT UP

Hark! the herald angels sing
Killem's pills are just the thing;
Peace on earth and mercy mild,
Two for man and one for child.
Traditional rhyme

Before you take his Drop or Pill,
Take leave of Friends, and make your Will.
"Of Quack Doctors,"
Grubstreet Journal, 1735

By the eve of the first settlement of America, the mountebank had invaded every corner of Europe with his tonics and elixirs. Operating at fairs, on street corners, in market squares, or wherever a crowd was likely to gather, the traveling quack quickly learned how to capitalize on the ordinary man's ignorance and simplicity, and on his fear of illness, pain, and death. In order to succeed as a street seller of medicine, or a corn cutter or tooth drawer, he was required not only to attract a crowd, but to hold it and convince some of its members that he possessed the power to relieve their real or fancied suffering.

Like his cousin the street conjurer, the mountebank depended on patter, misdirection, and confusion to establish power over the crowds that assembled at his stage. His prime objective was to keep the audience interested but uncritical; he required the spectators' attention, but not such close attention that the logic of his harangue would come under too careful scrutiny. Most mountebanks found the answer in a free show which combined their lecture with tricks, demonstrations, music, and comedy. The shows had absolutely nothing to do with the medicines, cheap soap, or smelling salts hawked by the doctor. But they were entertaining and distracting, and an excellent blind for the mountebank's real object, his sales pitch to the assembled crowd.[1]

Some quacks performed on the pavement or from a bench or table. The more prosperous carried a simple platform, which could be raised to head height on trestles or barrels, or a booth

Wallpaper detail, 1825: a quack and zanies on a stage. Deutsches Tapeten-Museum, Kassel. PHOTO COURTESY OF JAMES HARVEY YOUNG.

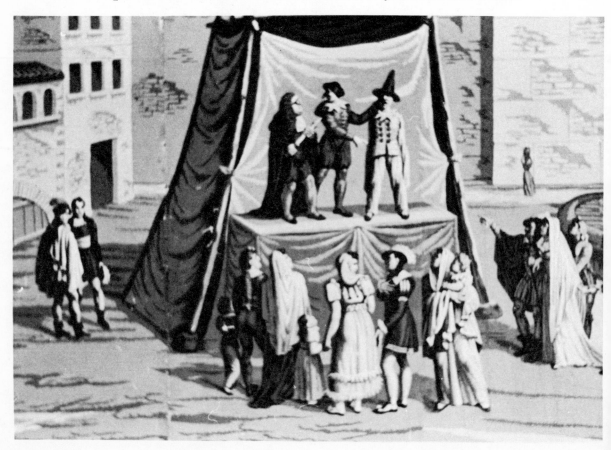

stage like those used by *commedia dell' arte* troupes and other strolling players. The booth arrangement provided a curtained-off area behind the stage which served the doctor as laboratory and consulting room. Inside he concocted his pills and syrups and treated those patients whose symptoms called for at least some measure of privacy; on the outdoor platform he pulled teeth, pared corns, and delivered his harangues while his servants dispensed drugs or entertained the crowd.

The performances of the famous mountebanks of Venice are typical of the sort of shows to be seen all over Europe by the seventeenth century. Every day half a dozen platforms were set up by quacks in the Piazza San Marco, and each morning and afternoon their owners loudly and urgently competed for the attention of the crowd. In preparation for his show, each doctor mounted his platform and busied himself with the contents of a gaudy medicine chest as his performers milled about, tuning their musical instruments and joking with the crowd. All this time, the doctor was keeping a watchful eye on the spectators; when he was satisfied that the moment was right, he signaled to his performers to begin the show. "After the whole rabble of them is gotten on the stage," wrote an English traveler, Thomas Coryat, "whereof some weare vizards being disguised like fooles in a play, some that are women (for there are divers also amongst them) are attyred with habits according to that person they sustaine; after (I say) they are all upon the stage, the musicke begins."[2]

As the music played, the quacking doctor opened his trunk and set out the vials of medicine that he hoped to peddle to the spectators. Then he began an oration, lasting half an hour or more, "wherein he doth most hyperbolically extoll the vertue of his drugs and confections . . . Though many of them are very counterfeit and false. Truly I often wondred at many of these naturall Orators. For they would tell their tales with such admirable volubility and plausible grace, even *extempore,* and seasoned with that singular variety of elegant jests and witty conceits, that they did often strike admiration into strangers that never heard them before: and by how much the more eloquent these Naturalists are by so much the greater audience they draw unto them, and the more ware they sell."

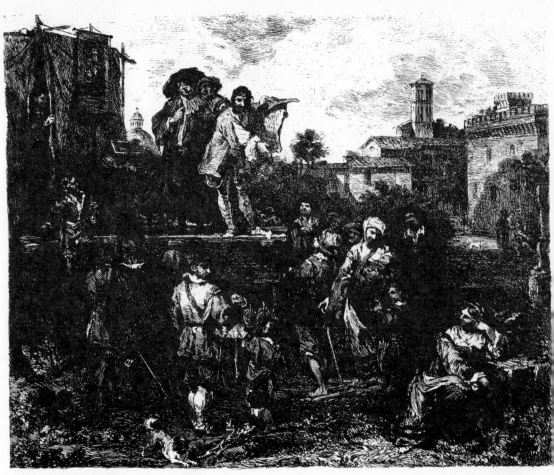

P. van Laar, *The Charlatan.*

PICTURE COLLECTION, NEW YORK PUBLIC LIBRARY.

The style and content of a mountebank's lecture varied with his tastes and inclinations: some specialized in blood-chilling recitals of the toll disease was taking on the assembled specta-tors. Orations of this sort, sometimes accompanied by sinister charts and jars of alcohol containing what passed for hideously diseased organs, presented the symptoms of fatal illness in such general terms that anyone with the slightest touch of hypochondria could easily feel himself only steps away from the grave. Other charlatans, of a less sober turn of mind, de-pended largely on extravagant rhetoric and airy patter to wear down the sales resistance of potential customers.[3] After the lecture and sale came more music, comedy and tricks, al-ternating with a second and perhaps a third lecture, and sales of drugs, perfumes, ballads, and cheap rosaries and holy pic-tures, until in the showman's judgment, every last penny had been squeezed from the dwindling crowd.

The free entertainment that accompanied the quack's harangue, like the design of his stage, was borrowed from the popular theatre of the day. Strollers of every sort—jugglers, conjurers, slack wire walkers, and strong men—attached themselves to the companies of the medicine showmen. In Italy and France a simple *commedia dell' arte* performance was often one of the inducements offered the crowd by the mountebank. It was the *zanni* or clowns of the *commedia* that proved most popular with audiences, and ultimately the clown figure (called a "Zany" or a "Merry Andrew" in England) became the quack's principal ally. At Wisbeach fair the eighteenth-century playwright Thomas Holcroft watched a zany parade through the streets with a drummer, drawing customers to his master's booth. When he had mustered a crowd, the zany leaped onto the stage, "alighting half upright, roaring with pretended pain, pressing his hip declaring he had put out his collar-bone, crying to his master to come and cure it, receiving a kick, springing

F. A. Maulpertsch, *The Charlatan*, 1785.

PICTURE COLLECTION, NEW YORK PUBLIC LIBRARY.

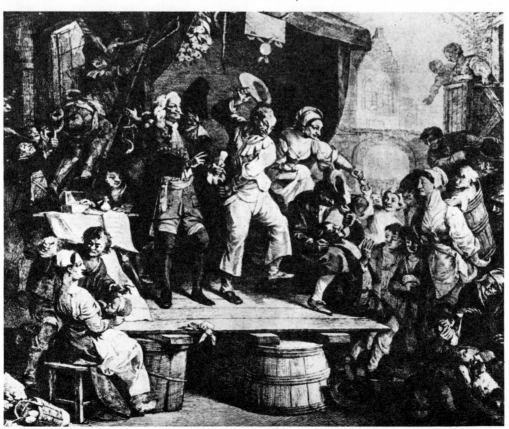

up and making a somersault; thanking his master kindly for making him well, yet the moment his back was turned, mocking him with wry faces; answering the doctor, whom I should have thought extremely witty, if Andrew had not been there with jokes so apposite and whimsical, as never failed to produce roars of laughter."[4] Some quacks and their zanies performed short plays in which the doctor played himself and the zany his unwilling patient.[5] Others exhibited snakes, giant lizards or Egyptian crocodiles to draw the curious to their booths, or spun eggs on a stick, danced with bowls of water on their heads, or performed acrobatic feats or magic tricks.[6] One observer spoke darkly of quacks who handled poisonous snakes by the hour or gashed their arms with knives and mysteriously healed them again.[7]

When the European quack and his zany entered the American colonies is not known. But early in the eighteenth century strolling acrobats, conjurers, animal trainers, and other cousins of the mountebank had become a common sight in every part of the colonies. Exhibitions of exotic animals competed for crowds with dwarfs, visiting Indian chieftains, and the Female Sampson, who "lies with her body extended between two chairs, and bears an anvil of 300 lb. on her breast, and will suffer two men to strike on it with sledge-hammers."[8] Along with the cheap showmen came an army of equally cheap medical practitioners. "Quacks abound like Locusts in *Egypt*," wrote William Smith in 1757, "and too many have recommended themselves to full Practice and profitable Subsistence. This is the less to be wondered at, as the Profession is under no Kind of Regulation . . . Any Man at his Pleasure sets up for Physician, Apothecary, and Chirurgeon."[9] Herb vendors wandered the streets with their baskets of wormwood, sassafras, sweet basil, mandrake, and rhubarb. Peddlers filled their packs and wagons with English patent tonics or nostrums which they bottled under their own labels.[10] Sincere but untrained laymen practiced medicine informally in out-of-the-way villages, and outright charlatans, many of them ignorant and dangerous, set up surgeries or made the rounds of country towns.[11] Soon the mountebank—half quack physician and half showman—had begun to hawk his wares from stages at fairs and court days.

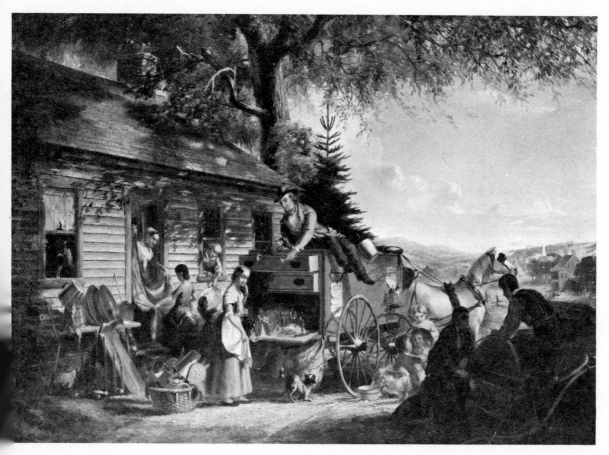

William H. Carlton, *The Pill Vendor.*

Before the Revolution performing quacks had become suf-
ficiently numerous that at least two colonies took pains to ban
their appearances. In 1772 New Jersey included a provision
aimed at mountebanks in an act regulating the practice of
medicine in the colony.[12] A year later Connecticut passed a
formidable "Act for suppressing of Mountebanks" that made
clear the official position of the colony toward idlers who
threatened the health and the morals of the unwary citizen:

> Whereas the practice of mountebanks in dealing
> out and administering physick and medicine of un-
> known composition indiscriminately to any persons
> whom they can by fair words induce to purchase and
> receive them without duly consulting, or opportunity
> of duly consulting, and considering the nature and
> symptoms of the disorder for which, and the constitu-

tion and circumstances of the patient or receiver to whom they administer, has a tendency to injure and destroy the health, constitution and lives of those who receive and use such medicines: And whereas the practice of mountebanks in publickly advertising and giving notice of their skill and ability to cure diseases, and the erecting publick stages and places from whence to declaim to and harangue the people on the virtue and efficacy of their medicines, or to exhibit by themselves or their dependents any plays, tricks, juggling or unprofitable feats of uncommon dexterity and agility of body, tends to draw together great numbers of people, to the corruption of manners, promotion of idleness, and the detriment of good order and religion, as well as to tempt and ensnare them to purchase such unwhole and oftentimes dangerous drugs:

Be it therefore enacted by the Governor, Council and Representatives, in General Court assembled, and by the authority of the same, That no mountebank, or person whatsoever under him, shall exhibit or cause to be exhibited on any publick stage or place whatsoever within this Colony, any games, tricks, plays, jugling or feats of uncommon decsterity and agility of body, tending to no good and useful purposes, but tending to collect together numbers of spectators and gratify vain or useless curiosity. Nor shall any mountebank, or person whatsoever under him, at or any such stage or place offer, vend or otherwise dispose of, or invite any person so collected to purchase or receive any physick, drugs, or medicines, commended to be efficacious and useful in various disorders.[13]

The somewhat more affluent and respectable acting troupes were frequently legislated against by town fathers, railed against from the pulpit, and shunned by conservative colonists. The mountebank, lacking even the doubtful refuge of a recognized place in the theatrical profession, was fair game everywhere and was to continue so long after other forms of theatre had gained at least some measure of respectability.

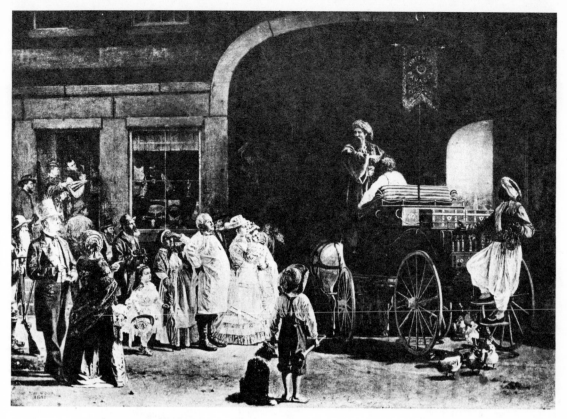

T. W. Wood, *The Quack Doctor*, 1882.

In spite of official opposition, the mountebank remained the delight of the crowd. A boatload of 120 men, women, and children voyaged from New York to Long Island in 1771 to see a strolling quack perform, and for their pains were shipwrecked on the voyage home.[14] John Brenon, a quack who passed through New York in 1787, offered a bountiful program to suffering and entertainment-starved New Yorkers: balloon ascensions; half a dozen tricks on the slack wire; singing and sleight of hand by Mrs. Brenon; a conjuring trick in which a member of the audience was invited to cut off the head of a fowl which Brenon would restore to life; and finally a miraculous cure for toothache "without drawing.—No cure, No pay. For the Poor Gratis."[15]

A simple show like that presented by Brenon and his wife was the staple of performing quacks for much of the nineteenth century. Traveling "doctors" and medicine peddlers, sometimes exotically garbed as Indians, Turks, or sorcerers, gathered crowds at court days and "protracted meetings" with magic,

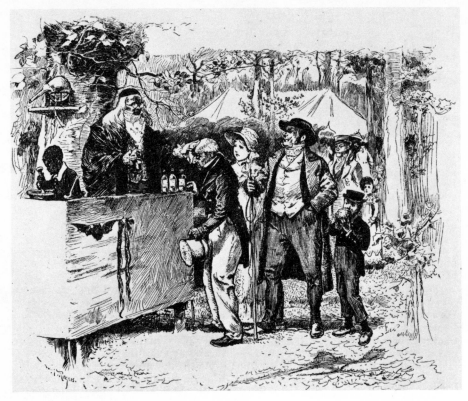

W. Rogers, *The Quack-Doctor*, 1889.

PICTURE COLLECTION, NEW YORK PUBLIC LIBRARY.

hypnotism, ventriloquism, or exhibitions of trick shooting. By the fifties, banjo tunes and blackface capers stolen from the minstrel show had been added, and on the eve of the Civil War some medicine men probably produced occasional performances of popular melodramas.[16] In most respects, however, the shows were not very different from the centuries-old performances of the European mountebanks. In Europe, as a matter of fact, there was to be little change in the traditional performing quack's show until the form died out early in the twentieth century. But by the seventies, the American patent medicine manufacturers, always in search of fresh ways to advertise their nostrums, had seized on the time-honored mountebank's performance and begun to reshape it to their own specifications.

The nineteenth century was a period of phenomenal growth in the American patent medicine industry. A wholesale drug catalogue issued in 1804 listed some eighty patent tonics; a catalogue that appeared in 1857 featured some 600, and in the following year a hydropathic physician was able to compile a list of more than 1,500 patent medicines.[17] Some of the men whose names and titles were attached to these tonics were honest physicians who had discovered and tested a preparation in which they genuinely believed. But others were simply former country peddlers who had discovered that patent medicines sold better than Yankee notions, or enterprising workmen who had developed a line of cures based on old family recipes. Not a few were ignorant and untrained quacks who guaranteed that their brews would cure "every disease, human and inhuman, between a hang-nail and natural death of two weeks standing."[18]

In his autobiography, P. T. Barnum quoted a French writer as saying: "The reader of a newspaper does not see the first insertion of an ordinary advertisement; the second insertion he sees, but does not read; the third insertion he reads; the fourth insertion he looks at the price; the fifth insertion he speaks to his wife; the sixth insertion he is ready to purchase; and the seventh insertion he purchases."[19] The patent medicine proprietors were among the first believers in Barnum's principle of advertising by inundation. Editors clenched their teeth and inserted the flood of advertisements. A few big newspapers, like Horace Greeley's New York *Tribune*, could afford the luxury of weeding out the most odious quack announcements. But many small-town and country papers devoted seemingly endless columns to obnoxious advertising because it was the only way to stay in business with a small circulation, and their columns were crammed with florid declarations of the amazing properties of Dr. Duponco's Golden Periodical Pills, Dr. Sappington's Vegetable Febrifuge Pills, or Dr. Hemmold's Genuine Preparation of Highly Concentrated Compound Fluid Extract of Buchnu.

Editors gained at least some small measure of revenge by flaying the patent medicine quacks in their columns. The archetypal quack, Dr. Balthasar Beckar—brassy, shrewd, and ignorant—was the creation of the editor of the Portsmouth (Ohio) *Journal* in 1824:

Dr. Balthasar Beckar respectfully informs the public, that he is possessed of the genuine ABRACADABRA and understands the true use of the Dandelion flowers.

He is the inventor of a PILL that will straighten a Roman nose into a Grecian; sharpen a bullet-nose to a keen edge; and bring down the most inveterate pug-nose to a reasonable degree of earthly mindedness. His DROPS are sovereign for all disorders of the teeth: they will extract the future decayed tooth from the gums of a nurse child, with intense delight, and will insert in lieu thereof a piece of polished ivory; they will give the breath any fragrance that the Patient may desire, and change the same at pleasure. Dr. *Balthasar Beckar* has a portable machine by which he frequently amuses himself with distilling rose water from his own breath. Onion-Eaters may be supplied with an apparatus for condensing their breath into Gum Assafoetida at a reasonable price. He has also a LOTION for converting the outer integuments into fur or broadcloath, at the will of the Patient.

The Unborn Doctor (for so Dr. Balthasar Beckar is commonly termed in the place of his nativity) scorns to make any professions which he is not able to fulfill.—As soon as the crowd of Patients will afford him a little leisure, he will endeavor to sell for publication a few of the certificates with which the gratitude of the world is continually loading the U. States' mail. His correspondence is immense, and he has the honor of having under his care at this moment several of the crowned heads of Europe.

N.B. Cancers cured by inspection. Boots and shoes cleaned and every favor gratefully acknowledged.

P.S. No cure, no pay.

** To prove the security of his professions, Dr. Balthasar Beckar will, on Monday next, precisely at 12 o'clock, standing on the pavement in front of the Athenaeum swallow one of his own Pills. Practitioners of Medicine, and men of science generally, and all others who are fond of philosophical experiments, are invited to attend and witness this heroic experiment.[20]

The advertisements of the real patent medicine proprietors were scarcely less fantastic. Many medicine men specialized in lugubrious testimonials from users of their products. "Miracle Cure," read the first line of an advertisement for the Dr. Williams Medicine Company of Schenectady, New York. The nature of the miracle was described in a testimonial letter from one Richard D. Creech of 1062 Second Street, Appleton, Wisconsin, whose son Willard had supposedly been completely paralyzed for nine months when a relative suggested a new medication. "In six weeks after taking the pills we noted signs of vitality in the legs, and in four months he was able to go to school," said the letter. "It was nothing else in the world that saved the boy but Dr. Williams Pink Pills for Pale People."[21] Others, like the redoubtable Lydia Pinkham, favored the high-minded parable, offering readers such snatches of homely wisdom as a piece under the heading "Who climbs too high, goes to fall," which dealt with nervous prostration in females and the role of Lydia E. Pinkham's Vegetable Compound in its prevention and cure.[22] Equally common were the advertisements that featured hair-raising scare techniques ("'Why Will Ye Die' When a never failing remedy for that dreadful scourge of Infancy and Childhood, the 'Croup' is at hand" or "DON'T DIE with the slow but sure-killing disease, Constipation"). The promoters of Mexican Mustang Liniment ("Foe of Pain, the Friend of Suffering Humanity, and the Salvation of the Patient, Toiling Brute") warbled their message to the tune of "Auld Lang Syne": "So long as human ills endure,/ And mortals suffer pain,/ So long shall MUSTANG LINIMENT/ Its glorious name maintain."[23]

Nostrum advertising continued to develop on a prodigious scale in nineteenth-century America: one promoter of a purgative was spending a hundred thousand dollars on various kinds of advertising at mid-century, and many of his competitors probably spent as much.[24] Along with newspaper advertisements, a sea of handbills, posters, flyers, free magazines,

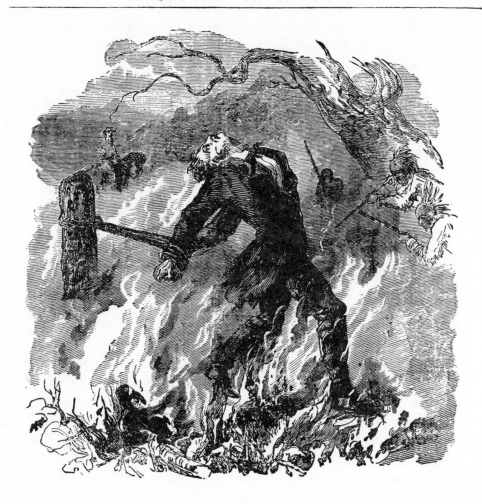

Burnt at the Stake!

HORRIBLE to behold, dreadful to relate! but don't waste a tear over such a wretch as Johnson Harris—that was his real name, but he had for many years had as many aliases as he had had residences. Crooked in his every action he came into existence warped to do evil and take advantage of his fellow man. If he ever had a good impulse it was when he turned his back on civilization; he sought the frontier, resolved to begin a new life and "turn over a new leaf."

The leaf was never turned, except to renew the same old pages of iniquitious criminality. There was much lawlessness on the frontier, and Johnson Harris only followed his natural bent when he allied himself with the lawbreakers. So grasping and over-reaching was the man, that he was not even that strange paradox—an honest thief, failing to deal fairly with his accomplices, until all along the border he was scorned alike by the false and true, neither honest man or rogue would countenance him.

In fear of the law, the miscreant dared not return to the States; with a healthy fear of Judge Lynch and the revenge of his former comrades in crime, he with a desperation born of despair and a desire to punish his enemies, allied himself to the Indians, and joined one of the wildest and fiercest tribes of the plains.

Rioting in bloodshed he made his name famous and infamous all along the border, until justly or unjustly he was accused of betraying his red allies and conspiring to betray them into the power of their greatest enemy, a rival tribe with whom they were frequently at war. Rightly or wrongly, so charged his presence and influence, had long aroused jealousy in the ranks of the savages and the outlaws, the infamous desperado perished at the stake, roasted alive!

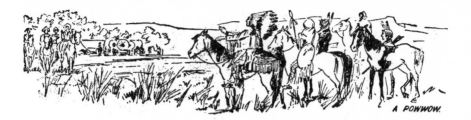

A POWWOW.

Exasperating Eczema Entirely Eradicated.

Sagwa Caused Complete Recovery.

Fall River, Mass.

For more than four years I had a chronic and very stubborn case of eczema and a great 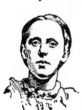 many even pronounced it blood poisoning. My feet and limbs were one mass of sores that all physicians and medicines failed to cure. Being almost discouraged I was at last induced to use *Kickapoo Indian Sagwa*. At first I was not satisfied with their actions but your agent insisted on my continuing in their use and I am more than thankful as now I am entirely cured, and wish all my friends and neighbors to know that the *Kickapoo Indian Sagwa* was the cause of my complete recovery.

GERTRUDE WALLBANK.

He Dismissed the Doctors.

Saved Expenses and Saved His Life.

Pawtucket, Rhode Island.

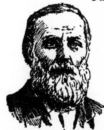 I was under the care of a doctor when I began to use *Kickapoo Indian Sagwa* for general debility. I dismissed him because the *Sagwa* did me more good than all the doctors. I can recommend it as the best medicine I know of. Friends of mine have used it by knowing what condition I was in before using *Sagwa*. They tried it for kidney and liver diseases and as a blood medicine and are all agreed; it is the best medicine they ever used and cannot praise it too highly.

TILLINGHAST S. MOWERY,
12 West Avenue.

Complication of Disorders.
Sagwa Wins Again.

Eastport, N. Y.

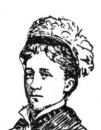 For the past five years I have been troubled with nervous prostration. I had loss of memory, weak heart, causing extreme palpitation, was constantly tired and obliged to lie down much of the time. I had loss of appetite and was terribly distressed by what little food I could eat. I finally commenced using *Kickapoo Indian Sagwa*, and immediately began to improve. My nerves were soon entirely strengthened, my food did not distress me and I was entirely cured. I cordially recommend *Sagwa* to all.

MRS. CHARLES H. GORDON.

Kickapoo Indian Oil.

His Never Failing Remedy.

Freeport, New York.

For some time I have been troubled with nervous headache and neuralgia so at times it 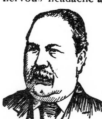 would seem as if I should go crazy. At last my mind was made up to try *Kickapoo Indian Oil*. Before I had used one bottle my head was much better. I have now started on a third bottle. The *Indian Oil* is my never-failing remedy. I am willing to testify to the good it has done in our family, with wonderful results.

THEODORE F. CORWIN.

trade cards, songsters, joke books, and almanacs poured from the presses of the patent medicine promoters.[25] By the seventies, some firms had begun to try out the ancient mountebank's show as a method of advertising and selling their medicines. And with that Barnumesque talent for the novel and flamboyant that marked the rest of their advertising, they began to transform the simple performance of the mountebank into a patent medicine extravaganza.

The medicine shows cheerfully borrowed everything that was taking place elsewhere in the American theatre. In the interests of Herbs of Joy or Ka-Ton-Ka, the Great Indian Medicine, vacant lots and village halls began to be filled with free plays, vaudeville, musical comedy, minstrels, magic, burlesque, dog and pony circuses, Punch and Judy shows, pantomime, menageries, pie-eating contests, and early motion pictures. Soon medicine shows carried companies of thirty-five or forty, sometimes moved by special train, owned enough canvas to outfit a small circus, and often drew crowds in the thousands on a pleasant summer night.

Before the turn of the nineteenth century the traveling medicine show, like the circus, the minstrel show, and the tent repertoire company, was a flourishing form of entertainment. Some medicine shows played New York, Boston, and Chicago with considerable success. But their natural home was a village square or a small-town opera house, and the medicine showman's favorite audience a crowd of eager rustics. Business was good: for many rural Americans the medicine show provided the only taste of professional entertainment from one year to the next, and showmen were not slow to capitalize on the possibilities. Small independent troupes and lone pitchmen, handling their own concoctions or such standard remedies as Lydia E. Pinkham's Vegetable Compound or Ayer's Sarsaparilla vied for audiences with companies sent out by such big firms specializing in medicine show advertising such as the Hamlin Company of Chicago, makers of Wizard Oil, and the famous Kickapoo Indian Medicine Company of New Haven.

By World War I the shows were no longer so vital a part of small-town life. The Model T and the motion picture were creating a new kind of audience that was increasingly less

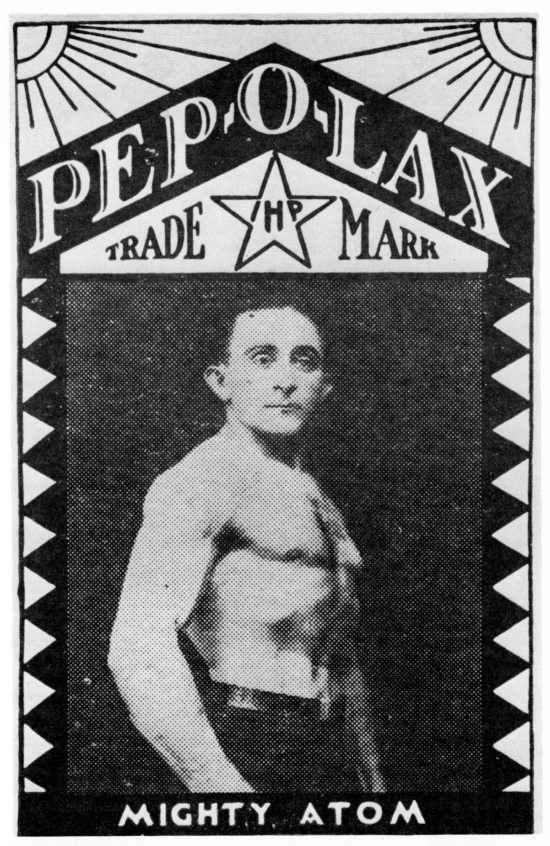

PEP·O·LAX

TRADE MARK

MIGHTY ATOM

Herb tonic box.   COLLECTION OF THE AUTHOR.

impressed by a Kickapoo war dance or the warblings of a
Wizard Oil Concert Company, and showmen found their audiences beginning to melt away. At the same time, new and
more stringent regulations concerned with manufacture and
labeling made the patent medicine business less profitable and
more difficult to operate. Each spring fewer shows started out
on the road, and by World War II the medicine showman,
though he still existed in a few remote areas, was virtually for-
gotten by most of the towns that had welcomed him half a
century before. Perhaps two dozen medicine show troupes continued to struggle along through the forties, and by 1964 the
last of the big shows had played its final performance.[26] At
least one old medicine pitchman, The Mighty Atom, still per-
forms feats of strength and lectures on health at fairs and
farmers' markets in the East, but the medicine show as a type
of popular entertainment has vanished—the victim, in large
part, of radio and television, the forms that it helped to
create.[27]

2

PITCHMEN, HIGH AND LOW

Where, oh, where are Big Foot Wallace, Dr.
Fraser, Doc. Murray, Dirty Dick Sullivan, Smooy
Bill, Comanche Charlie, Ivory Soap Ben, Big
Jim Hamilton, Red Nelson, Bedford Frenchy,
Doc. Trumble, and the other star pitchmen of
the olden days?

Dr. Bullywat,
"When High Pitchmen Had Brains"

At the turn of the nineteenth century the street worker or
pitchman was to be found in every American city. Descended
from the street sellers of drugs and ointments who arrived
with the first colonists, and a close cousin to the mountebank of
Europe, he generally worked alone or with a partner, loudly
hawking his medicines or novelties at busy intersections or on
vacant lots and fairgrounds. Unlike the medicine show proprietor, who created a full-scale show by alternating medicine
pitches and entertainment, the street worker—even though he
might travel with a banjo player or a blackface comedian—
depended chiefly on bits of music or comedy to draw a crowd
and on his bold and colorful patter to hold it.[1] Street work
could be lucrative for a skillful talker, but by the twenties and

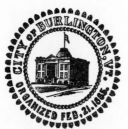

Burlington, Vt., *Aug. 9* 19*5 2*

RECEIVED FROM *A. W. Lithgow*

Two ———————————— **Dollars**

Deposited with his application for a LICENSE under

the City Ordinances for *Selling liniament*

from *One Day* to *Aug 9, 1922*

$ *2*

Edward B. Corley

City Clerk

Pitchman's license.   WILLIAM H. HELFAND COLLECTION.

thirties increasingly rigid laws against open-air peddling began
to drive the pitchman into less dangerous fields, and by the
mid-fifties he had virtually disappeared from the streets for
good.

In the rather rigid caste system of the medicine show world,
pitchmen were often looked down upon by the performers and
lecturers connected with the shows. The street workers, a former medicine showman wrote, were "regarded by the legitimate medicine men as being lower than a snake. There was
all the difference in the world between a medicine man and a
pitchman, who carried his slum in a satchel, ran like hell
when he saw an approaching cop and rarely returned to the
same place twice."[2] In actual fact the difference was not always
so plain. Most medicine showmen were prepared to present a
street-corner pitch when cash was short, and many alternated
between street work and work on the regular medicine show
companies. In the winter many small troupes were cut down in
size to save on expenses, and the doctor and a single musician
would set up a pitch at a farmers' market or tobacco market,
grinding away hour after hour with some simple combination
of music, lecture, and sale.[3] The professional pitchman, how-

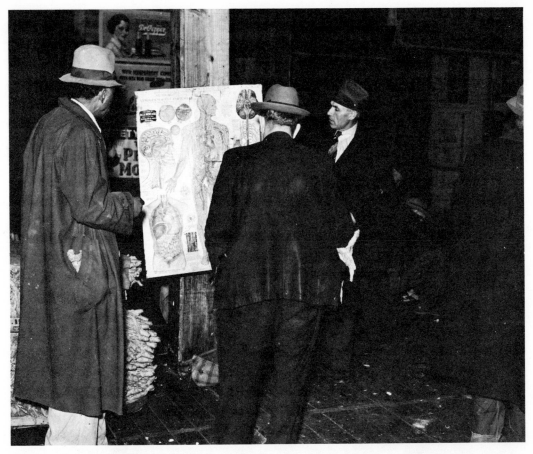

Pitchman giving a sales talk to farmers, Durham, North Carolina, 1940.   PHOTO BY POST. LIBRARY OF CONGRESS.

ever, was often viewed somewhat warily by the medicine show owner. Medicine pitchmen and showmen were linked in the public mind, and the pitchman, because of his mobility, was prone to the sort of irresponsibility and shady dealing that often gave all medicine sellers a bad name.

Among the street workers themselves, the high pitchman, who worked from a platform or the back of a wagon, was considered a superior being. A high pitch medicine man, wrote Violet McNeal, "belonged to the aristocracy of the pitch world."[4] As a member of the high pitch fraternity Miss McNeal scorned other kinds of street workers and refused to be seen with carnival people or circus performers. "It was permissible, however, to associate with circus owners. I could mingle with saloon owners, managers of gambling houses, race-horse owners, bookmakers, politicians, and high-class thieves, both men and women."[5] Farther down the social scale was the low pitch operator, who sold from a "tripes and keister" (a suitcase mounted on a tripod) in a doorway or on the sidewalk.[6]

Because they took trade out of town, street workers were always unpopular with established merchants. *Advertising World* fulminated against the pitchman who "sells more goods in half an hour than [the legitimate storekeeper] sells in a month."[7] "The street vendor," said the editors, "comes to town, opens up his pack, spends half an hour 'advertising' his stock orally, aided with a few sleight of hand tricks, a colored comedian, or a little slow music, and then proceeds to sell to your customers the very same goods you have had in your store for a month or more."[8] In spite of the hostility of local merchants, before the end of the nineteenth century licenses were relatively easy to obtain and generally inexpensive in many

Tripes and keister operator, Mebane, North Carolina, 1940.
PHOTO BY POST. LIBRARY OF CONGRESS.

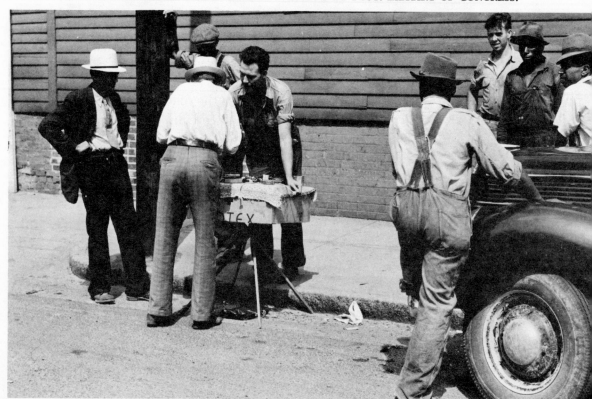

cities.[9] Increasingly, however, licenses (or "readers") became costly and difficult to purchase without bribing the police or a city official.

The welter of state, county and local licensing laws in some areas made it virtually impossible for a pitchman to make money unless he found a loophole. Some pitchmen made deals with local druggists, ostensibly operating their pitches as concessions for the drugstores, or, after World War I, carried a veteran who was entitled to special licensing privileges in certain localities.[10] Others simply did not pay. When Doc McBride played Stillwater, Minnesota, he balked at spending three dollars a day to pitch his King of Pain, and "departed in a huff, paid his bill at the Sawyer House, and left town with a great flourish of trumpets so to speak."[11] Milton Bartok, a high pitchman turned medicine showman, never bought licenses. "We used to pray for them to come on us for licenses, because we'd cause a big stink," said Bartok. "The medicine was my product, my own manufacture. I had an affidavit to that effect. So they'd come in and want a license, and I'd say 'No.' I'd want them to arrest me; then we'd buy pages in the newspapers and create the biggest stink you ever saw. You talk about rabble rousing . . . we'd have everybody in town down there to protect me—the good health evangelist."[12]

Until about World War I, pitchmen traveled in wagons pulled by horses or mules, or by rail, carrying their equipment in the baggage car.[13] The less fortunate used pack burros, hopped convenient freight trains, or sent their trunks ahead and walked the railroad tracks from one town to another.[14] After the war, pitchmen began more and more to travel by house-car—basically a truck adapted for eating and sleeping, with a tailgate that dropped down to form a tiny stage—or by automobile. One pitchman converted an open touring car into a moving high pitch platform by removing the cushions from the rear seat to create a solid base for his podium and setting up a huge umbrella for a backdrop.[15] Some late pitchmen rigged up ingenious electric lighting systems, but many continued to pitch by the light of the traditional gasoline torch, an object as much identified with the street worker as his banjo, his tripes and keister, and his top hat and black tailcoat.[16] Improvised torches were fashioned by the pitchman from a tomato can, a broomstick, some cotton, and a quantity of alcohol. More substantial "banjo" or "pan" torches were made by blacksmiths from a length of pipe to which was welded a gasoline reservoir and another shorter length of pipe fitted with a patent "Baker Burner."[17]

Once he had set up, the pitchman usually began with some sort of simple entertainment to draw the crowd (or "tip") to his pitch. Ventriloquism, jokes, magic, and banjo music were standard attention getters, and many pitchmen and small medicine showmen teamed up with buskers or "busters," the wandering singers who performed for coins in saloons, on the edge of carnivals, or outside mines and factories on paydays.[18] Some pitchmen, however, drew tips with more colorful and eccentric devices. Exotic animals were popular: monkeys were frequently used, along with an assortment of reptiles that included Gila monsters, lizards, alligators, and every sort of snake.[19]

A loathsome display of tapeworms coiled in jars of alcohol or formaldehyde—supposedly taken from the pitchman's customers, but probably purchased at a local stockyard—was the standard come-on of the tapeworm specialist.[20] Calculator Williams attracted customers with displays of lightning mathematics, and Milton Bartok began by seemingly burning money or igniting himself with a blowtorch.[21] Professor Ray Black developed an impressive scheme for drawing a crowd that centered around a length of rope, a Bible, and a human skull. In a town square or a vacant lot on a busy street, Black would lay out his strange properties, placing them on the ground next to his folding table and medicine case. Then he would begin, with painstaking care and concentration, to arrange and rearrange them. Apparently oblivious to the fascinated crowd that gradually gathered around him, Black would continue his curious work for half an hour or more until he was satisfied with the size of his tip. Then he would suddenly begin his medicine lecture, never once mentioning in it the Bible, rope or skull.[22]

The uninspired pitchman spoke badly and often illiterately, and usually delivered a mechanical-sounding stereotyped pitch. The bad lecturer, said Milton Bartok, would often work with a Bible, using a traditional pitch: "'The Bible says, "Roots, barks, herbs and berries"'—and blablabla!"[23] But in the case of a really first-rate lecturer, the pitch was an entertainment in its own right. A newspaper editor wrote fondly of "Leather-Lungs," a pitchman who took up a spot near the police station each year, where he presented "one of the greatest discourses ever delivered on the ills of mankind, the woes of the world, and the distressful condition of the universe," in a voice "that can be heard for several city blocks, around corners and through alleyways."[24] The best were skilled orators who never wearied an audience and were able to manipulate the emotions of a crowd like a good tent evangelist. "You could feel if your story was being received," said Bartok. "When you were talking to a big crowd it was like fighting a big fish. You could feel that they were your people. You would get on your toes—literally—working. You would come down from there ringing wet. It was a feeling you got, a sort of vibration you got from the people."[25] Bartok saw some danger in being too articulate before a crowd, however, and he cultivated an intentionally hesitant style to avoid the label of the confidence man and to allow young people to translate for their parents and grandparents in areas where little English was spoken.[26] "The smooth talkers put the people on guard," Bartok said. "'He's a sharpie; he's a smooth talker'—once you hear that you're done."[27]

When a number of pitchmen gathered together in one place the effect was impressive. A lot favored by pitchmen in Los Angeles became a kind of bizarre street fair, featuring Prince Nanzetta and Arizona Bill, both appropriately costumed, selling medicine, along with other street workers handling flea powder, razor-strop dressing, spot remover, soap, and Gummy-Ga-Ho, the pitchman's traditional cheap cement for repairing broken china and furniture. One pitchwoman sold chameleons, and there was a mummy on exhibition and the traditional carnival snake pit.[28] The pages of *The Billboard*, the magazine most widely read by pitchmen and medicine showmen, were filled with the advertisements of wholesalers of shoddy rings, watches, fountain pens, combs, wallets, belts, neckties, and such intriguing novelties as the Gaso-Phone, to be installed in Fords and Chevrolets, which rang when the fuel supply had dropped to one gallon.[29] In fact, a pitchman's head could be turned by any product, no matter how bizarre, that appeared to be a potential money-maker. But the favorites with most pitchmen were cheap novelties of all kinds, drugs and corn cures, soap, and so-called electric belts and liver pads. A number of street workers were tooth-pulling specialists, practicing what passed for painless dentistry in many rural communities.

The pitchman's staple was the herb compound, made up of various vegetable substances and purporting to have tonic and cathartic qualities. Although most herb remedies tended toward the innocuous, those sold before the Food and Drugs Act of 1906 were often extravagantly described on boxes and labels and in street workers' pitches as "sure cures" for a fantastic range of diseases. The usual herb tablets or liquid sold for about a dollar before World War I, and were often pitched along with a liniment for fifty cents, a salve at twenty-five cents, a catarrh cure or corn remedy at ten cents, and a soap at ten cents or three for a quarter.

A number of pitchmen dealt only in corn remedies or soap. The Herb Remedy Company of Blair, Nebraska, advised "Agents, Streetmen, Medicine Men" that "if your bank roll is not sufficient to carry you through the long winter months," it could be replenished quickly by selling Magic Wonder Ointment for the feet.[30] The ointment might be transported in an intriguing product of the American Papier Mâché and Cotillon Works, "a special papier mâché foot 18″ long that has received numerous recommends. This is cast hollow that your wares may be carried inside and the same is built in true conformity as to lines etc. with a regular foot."[31] As in the case of most products sold by street workers, things were seldom what they seemed. Henry Gale peddled a corn ointment that was largely collodion, which has little effect on corns, and Doc Ruckner sold a preparation that was made from gasoline, camphor gum, and sassafras.[32] On the platform he "cured" corns through the shoes of volunteers—the gasoline soaking through the leather producing a soothing but quite temporary coolness in the area of the aching corn.[33]

When it comes to fixing, though, the laurels go to Henry Stahl, who, when the little town of Brookville, Pa., was crowded and the space at a premium, grabs both space and a room. He fixed the privilege man. Tell us how you did it, Henry.

Somebody said: "No one worked in Buffalo last Friday." Mutt Gordon had to lay off to register." Is Buffalo open? Do you vote there?

Hillsdale Mich., isn't what it was. Gravy for the home guard but the knight gets a swift kick. Ask Jack Goodwin, he knows.

HORNS
By Hornburger

Sand is great stuff, but don't get an eyeful. There is some hope for the wrongdoer who has a sign on his face. There is no crime in being human, but this is ofttimes translated as being an easy mark. To give is nobler than to receive—this refers especially to a black eye. Booze is great stuff! It makes some see snakes, others stars, and some imagine they are stars.

Wonder what Blake Burns, Flannagan and Culliton were looking for on East street in Raleigh, N. C., with that lantern?

Detroit Murphy was working slangs and supers in Michigan last year, and cleaning up, incidentally, when suddenly he bent over and whispered in a bystander's ear: "Did you get yours?" And the umpchay came right back: "Yessiree, young feller; you got me last year."

Gilman worked a big one at Saginaw, Mich., and sold out in two days, and rushed home to wifey in Detroit. Gilman is a hard worker.

The rumor is afloat that Billy Goodwin has consolidated with Kresge, Woolworth and the Kreses. Billy is getting in so much stock that you can hardly edge around the store. Mutt Gordon, shoot him a line.

A. G. Deifendorf—The boys at 324 Clark want to hear from you.

Bill Culliton and Snookum Flanagan, after a week's rest at the N. H. resort, jumped to Raleigh, N. C., and report big business.

A. L. Pierce, with a fine display of green goods, did a land-office business at Raleigh, N. C.

Miner sure passed out the sticks at Columbia, S. C.

Wm. Burns at Fayetteville, S. C., is doing nicely with solder.

Among the notables collecting on the sheet at Columbia, S. C., are: D. Lee Phune, Martin, Frank Flynn, Robbins, Mac Vean, Mark and Anthony, and all had time for auto rides after dark.

Poe McLean says that remarking about his pretty Okay gets him mad, but there's other things that get him madder.

What's doing this winter, Joe Krause?

For a day and night grinder hat's off to Mr. Reiss.

Craig, with the jar wrench and a good stand at Columbia, S. C., was contented after the fair was over.

Cincinnati has been the spot for surprises the past week: The little Doc Moran has returned to the fold of the faithful never looking better; Jack Crawford, dressed like a Christmas tree, was another, and our good friends, Mr. and Mrs. Al Reed, of gummygahoo fame, dropped in on us looking fine and feeling better. Al says he may stick around the Queen City for a while and then head for the land of cotton. Becker blowed to Vincennes, and it is said that the Southern gentleman, Joe Wilson, has opened a store in Cincy, but this has not been confirmed. Bill Shadell is still with us and looking fine.

Will Reiss, with everything under the sun, had the crowds digging deep all the time.

Fine weather and crowds make a man work like hell.

Bob Peyser, with forms, entertains the rubes at the Southern Fairs.

One thing is certain—that you are never too tired at night to count up.

Owing to poor health Hugh Duffy walked from New Hampshire to Erie, Pa.

Wonder why Buck Turner, of Washburn's Shows, does not like the wild girls?

If you have a business proposition to offer offer it in a business-like way, and your chances of success are improved 100 per cent.

George Gray, of hoopla fame, is not enjoying good health at present.

Old Big-foot Wallace says it's a bit lonesome at St. Joe, and wants some of his old friends to drop him a line once in a while. His address is F. G. Wallace, Lock Box 1268, St. Joseph, Mo.

H. R. Cox, Sta. 23, Detroit, wants to know where he can get the white slave books.

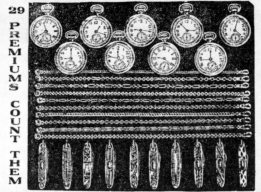
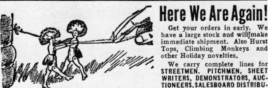

A few of the jam workers are doing nice work—that's why Spartanburg, S. C., is floating a century reader.

No matter how high the spite fence is the other fellow can think over it.

S. Herman and Billy Berger spent a week lay-off at the Oklahoma State Fair with the X on H. B., waiting for the Hot Springs doings. Sam got guy and annexed a pump crutch, and Billy Berger spoiled the celebration with a Charley Chaplin. They would like to hear from Shorty Lacoff, of picture fame. Write 'em care The Billboard.

And Robert Hilliard Walker, the doctor of corns—where have you seen him?

Doc Copeland is doing his little card tricks and passing out the celebrated tobacco cure for four bits. He is playing a little tune on one of Max Glusberg's tin lizzies at the opening every night. Doc is still in the Mormon State.

Hey, fellers, look who's here: Mike Crouch has been playing around in New York for the past couple months and says he's going nice, but the infantile paralysis scare did some damage.

A corn doctor was giving a demonstration in a New York town. He invited a chap who had a very painful corn on the stand to be treated. In doing this he knocked a box over on the doctor's foot. Doc grabbed his foot in his hand and danced around on one leg, hollering, "Gee, my corn!" The crowd laughed, and if he hadn't said he was fooling the ointjay would have been jimmed.

Which reminds us that Doc Dodge has come to the front with a new project which he says will be a winner—if it works. He wants to start an aeroplane ferry across the Niagara Falls. He says that filling the bag with Dodge corn dope, and shaped like his bottles, would carry it Okay.

Trixi Amlin is back in musical comedy again.

P. H. Holcombe, from down Tennessee, says he will be back, and soon. He speaks of B. J. Lindsay, who died recently from injuries received in a brawl in Greenwood, Miss. P. H. says there was no more inoffensive man than Lindsay, and he is strongly of the opinion that it was a case of town bully and stranger.

Doc V. Edward Curtis made Bassett, Neb., last week and cleaned up. He said it was the biggest of the season for him.

Harry Maier wants to hear from Mac Berkson.

Charlie Kost died July 29 at Columbus, O., from tuberculosis. He was buried in the family plot at Greenfield, O.

Frank Watts, care the Bexar Co. Hospital, Southton, Tex., who has been sick for the past three years would like to hear from his friends.

Vaseline Joe Ackerman reports as being the only representative of the noble order of Knights of the Tripod in Omaha. On peelers and sharpeners Joe says biz is good.

B. C. Blake, with aluminum solder, made a jump from Nashua, N. H., to Raleigh. But it pays.

G. D. Newport or any one knowing his address, have him wire his mother at Seneca, Ill., as she is very ill.

Mrs. Tommy Styner—Tommy's in a hurry to hear from you. Shoot him a line care the Electric Appliance Co., Burlington, Kan.

It looks like Happy Jack Marichal has deserted the cause for keeps, as he is perfectly happy and making a bunch of bucks with a car-py-val.

Charley Tryon is still in K. C., but he doesn't think much of the city.

Some class to Ernie or rawther B. R. Proctor, for he's a business man now. The Proctor Rug and Carpet Co., Ltd. (Ernie says he refers to the B. R.), now located in Butte Mont., permanently, and he's not hanging out the sign as a grubbery to the gang, but all his old friends will be welcomed. Ernie says this life is a case of outs and ins all the time. If he doesn't look out he won't have a look in, etc. We'll join the bunch and wish him all the luck in the world, so that when he'll be out he'll be "in," and not in when he's "out."

R. W. Lamb, that enterprising fiscal agent (new name—a rose by any other name, etc.), has landed on his list, The Daily Oklahoman, and says they won't be able to handle the circulation. R. W. likes big figures. Good luck!

In New Orleans right now: Andy Watson, working the old reliable pacerine, and the Missus, working pens; Mr. and Mrs. Levy, W. P. Danker and wife and Sam Storch—more to follow.

Nope, the story's all wrong Doc Simms isn't dead—merely fell and broke his leg, and is laid up at the Almac Hotel at St. Louis. He wants to hear from a few of the burglars.

Advertisements from *The Billboard*, 1916.

Most shows and many street workers sold soap along with their patent medicines, often pitching it first to help warm up a crowd for the more expensive herb remedies or liniments.[34] Many pitchmen were exclusively "soap workers." Their small foil-wrapped squares, which ordinarily cost no more than two cents apiece and sold from ten cents to a quarter, were ordered from supply houses or merely cut from large bars of laundry soap and encased in the soap worker's personal wrappers.[35] Soap was a favorite among pitchmen because it aroused less curiosity among druggists and physicians who might cause trouble than did patent medicines, and because the sale of soap required more brass than capital. Charlie White, the originator of White's White Wonder soap, found himself almost broke in Omaha, Nebraska, after a long stretch of rainy weather. His total assets consisted of his white broadcloth suit and white silk hat, five gross of soap, and a ten-dollar bill. "I paid three dollars to get the suit cleaned and the hat blocked," said White. "I paid two dollars for a license. I hired a white horse, hitched to a cream colored buck-board, paying three dollars in advance. I drove to a street corner and gave a boy the last two dollars to get me a pitcher of water—and the 'flash' of that two dollars for a simple errand sold over three gross of that soap, at twenty-five cents each, in two hours. That night I ordered another five gross of soap, together with salve and liniment, and with the aid of a colored banjo player and singer, I averaged a little over $100.00 a day for the next four weeks in Omaha."[36]

"They travel with all large Tent Shows, Carnivals, Midways, and Street Fairs," said an advertisement that described the soap worker's calling. "They are at Seaside Resorts and Watering Places wherever there are large gatherings. They show it up, Shampoo Heads, Clean Teeth, Make Pyramids of Lather, Blow Soap Bubbles and TALK SOAP."[37] Some talked it with special ingenuity. Silk Hat Harry—who drew crowds with card and rope tricks and peddled a soap that carried his picture, complete with identifying topper—used a pitch which contrasted the impurities found in ordinary soaps with his own remarkable "cleansing compound made of pure vegetable and edible oils such as coconut oil, palm oil, oil from flowers, and

Herb tonic box.

whites of eggs, saponified with soap bark that grows in the highest altitudes of Colorado."[38] In order to demonstrate that his cleansing agent contained "no poisons, acids, dead dogs, cats, or other dead animals," Harry ended his oration by cheerfully munching a cake of soap.[39] A rival soap worker, Doc Ruckner, dipped his hands in lather, which he allowed to dry on his skin before he mounted the lecture platform. When he washed his hands onstage, a mountain of suds overflowed the basin, offering a powerful testimony to the miraculous cleaning power of whatever soap Ruckner happened to be peddling.[40]

The nineteenth century was obsessed with the vital necessity of keeping the liver in good repair.[41] "The Great Organ," read the headline of one testimony to the importance of the liver: "Not the one in Boston or Philadelphia, but one vastly larger. The two mentioned are heard only occasionally, and then by a few thousand people; but the one we allude to is in action every minute of the day and concerns every human being all over the world. Need we remind you that we have reference to the liver? This is the largest gland or organ in the human body, and on it depends the health of the person owning it."[42] The liver pad was a consistent best seller. The formulas varied: Percy Williams, a medicine man who later became an important vaudeville manager, filled his version with a mixture of bran, mustard, hydrastis, and fenugreek while the firm of Flagg and Healy, it is reported, stuffed their pads with sawdust.[43] In both cases the single vital ingredient was capsicum—red pepper. Flagg and Healy customers were admonished to place a red spot on the pad directly over the liver. The spot was a mixture of red pepper and glue which melted at body temperature and spread a warm glow of what appeared to be returning health through the afflicted area.[44]

The electric or galvanic belt was a street-corner and mail-order best-seller that rivaled the liver pad in popularity. Fraser's Electric Catarrh Cure produced a tidy fortune for its proprietor, and Doc William Mosely, an unusually clever pitchman for Percy Williams's German Electric Belt who called himself "Electric Bill from over the hill," proudly pointed out that he "never worked and never will."[45] Fraser, Mosely, and the

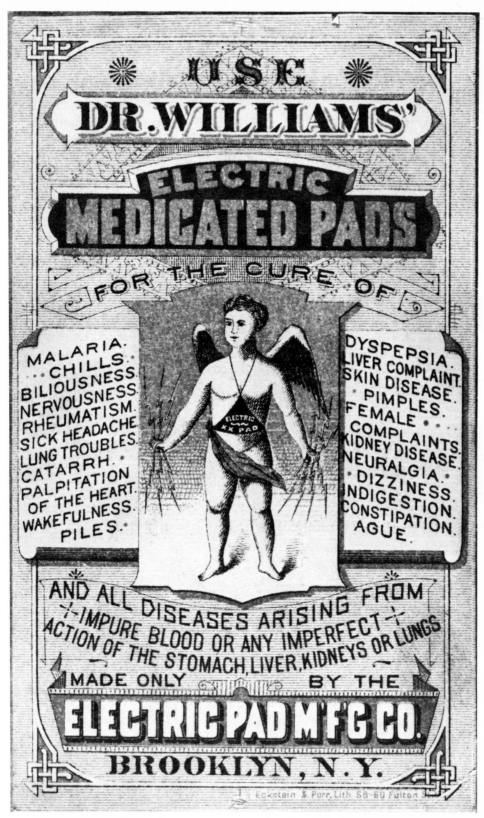

Liver pad trade card.

other electric pitchmen succeeded largely because the late nineteenth century remained somewhat hazy about the medical properties of electricity. Nolan's Famous Electric Catarrh Cure promised "fifty thousand volts of electricity confined in a two drachm bottle, yet harmless and powerful to do good," and a traveling dentist pulled teeth—supposedly "without pain and without charge"—as a result of his miraculous discovery of Electric Ozone.[46] The connection of these remedies and devices with electricity was remote if not totally nonexistent. Like the ubiquitous liver pad, the principal ingredient of most electric belts was usually red pepper, most often used to saturate a strip of felt studded with tin disks painted to simulate zinc and copper electrodes.[47] Big Foot Wallace featured an improved model covered in purple satin with zinc disks soaked in vinegar which produced a short-lived "electric" tingle.[48] The belts, usually sold for "the relief of sciatica and backache," were to be "worn around the naked torso during the hours of slumber," and presumably produced a machine-gun-like rattle each time the sufferer moved in his sleep.[49]

For many ordinary people at the turn of the nineteenth century, the only answer to an aching molar often lay in a much postponed trip to one of the cheap "dental parlors" to be found in most cities, or resort to one of the traveling tooth pullers who provided free entertainment to distract the wary or the cowardly from his principal business.[50] The so-called dental parlors were usually little more than factories for tooth extraction and the lowest grade of dental work. In New York City they were everywhere. Five thousand unlicensed dentists were to be found in the city in 1916, many of them either running or in the employ of cheap dental offices like those operated by the king of quack dentistry, Dr. "Painless" Parker.[51] The approach to advertising used by such practitioners was direct and colorful. One Dr. Hill, a Charlotte, North Carolina, "painless" dentist, set up billboards showing a maiden, pursued by a gigantic devil with forceps in his hand, beneath the legend, "Old Way of Pulling Teeth." Under the title, "Dr. Hill's Way," the same maiden, wearing a radiant and perfect smile, sat next to the Doctor himself, who held up for all to see her painlessly extracted tooth.[52] The redoubtable Parker used signs 20 feet high by 110 feet long, which ran around the second stories of various New York buildings, proclaiming, "Painless Parker—I am positively IT in painless dentistry!" Each "IT" was a full four stories high, and Parker once speculated that they were visible from four miles away.[53]

The carnival atmosphere associated with dental parlor advertising was a reflection on the whole spirit of painless dentistry as it was practiced on the road, by independent tooth extractors. Nevada Ned Oliver once played against a formidable husband and wife team of tooth pullers at the city market in Baltimore. Madame de Bois (sometimes known as Madame du Plat) and her husband, Dr. Andrew Dupré, pulled teeth and sold liniment to the accompaniment of a small brass band. Dupré was an extraordinary character who dressed in the uniform of a French chasseur, complete with doeskin breeches and a tall horsehair helmet. The hilt of his sword contained a forceps which he used to draw teeth as the band played "tooth-pulling music" to drown the screams of his customers.[54] A variation on the usual musical accompaniment to dentistry was devised by a Professor Seguar, an American healer who toured England in the early years of the twentieth century. Dressed in an eccentric Western outfit with a broad-brimmed sombrero, the Professor would pitch his Seguar's Oil and Prairy Flower Mixture, and then proceed to open his "dental clinic" in a tiny cabin built on the back of his carriage. As he moved into the cabin with each victim, Professor Seguar lit a miner's lamp on his giant headpiece and his band struck up the Negro spiritual, "Who's dat callin' so sweet?"[55]

Diamond Kit, a painless dentist who sported coat buttons set with rhinestones, a gigantic zircon tiepin, and a shining crown of glass diamonds on the top of his pillbox cap, worked from the back of a rented buggy. Like tooth pullers of all times, he began by arranging a formidable display of dentists' instruments, even though during his open-air operations he used nothing but a pair of simple extraction forceps. When a crowd had gathered, drawn by the jewelry, the pan torches tied to the wheels of his buggy, and the glittering dental equipment, Diamond Kit began his stock dental lecture. Kit's career as a dentist, he told audiences, had begun when he discovered by accident his miraculous Painkiller. So fantastic was the power of Diamond Kit's Painkiller that he was willing to demonstrate it as a public service without cost to the spectators or the lucky sufferer who volunteered to have a tooth drawn in public. After swabbing the victim's mouth with Painkiller, Kit brandished his forceps, grabbed the patient around the head with his hand across the windpipe—thus cutting off any agonized screams—and deftly extracted the offending tooth. Immediately after the extraction, Kit jammed a huge wad of cotton into the patient's mouth and asked him for his opinion of the operation. The muffled grunts of agony that were delivered in response were interpreted as an expression of admiration for Diamond Kit's work as a painless tooth extractor.[56]

There was always a considerable amount of lighthearted fraud involved with the products and services offered by pitchmen. But the vast majority stopped short of the most blatant forms of dishonesty. "Out on the streets I cin tell More lise then Patch hell a Mile," said a medicine man about his customers, but "I cant lie to them When thay set clos to Me."[57] There were those, however, to whom the face-to-face lie was a basic tool of the trade. To the so-called "jamb" or "jam" pitchman, there were no nice distinctions between pitching and confidence games. Shortchanging, forced sales, and dangerous misrepresentation of drugs marked the jamb worker's transactions with his customers, many of whom came to loathe all pitchmen as a result of an especially painful experience with

Quack's advertisement.   COLLECTION OF THE AUTHOR.

a jamb worker. Although a number of "legitimate" pitchmen turned jamb man from time to time when especially hard pressed for money, the jamb worker was generally disliked and distrusted by more scrupulous street workers for the "trail of closed towns, exorbitant licenses and public suspicion" that followed in his wake.[58]

The archetypal jamb pitchmen was Big Foot Wallace, a former rural schoolteacher whose real name was Frank White.[59] About 1880 White gave up teaching and acquired his new name, probably as a result of reading John C. Duval's *The Adventures of Big-Foot Wallace, the Texas Ranger and Hunter.*[60] The original Wallace, who lived until 1899, was something of a folk hero late in the nineteenth century, well known through Duval's book for his genial eccentricity and his extravagant sense of humor.[61] White, the new Big Foot Wallace, was a match for his namesake in every way—he was the street worker extraordinary, described by *The Billboard* as a "natural-born pitchman and a genius."[62] Wallace's talents resulted in the creation of elaborate confidence tricks and hard-sell jamb pitches, among them his blood bitters pitch, during which he would point a gigantic revolver at the crowd and solemnly intone: "Friends, listen to me. If I were the father of a family and one of my children were sick, and a man came to my town selling medicine, and I bought it for my sick child, and that man lied to me, he'd climb, neighbors, and he'd climb the tallest tree he could find, for I would shoot him like I would shoot a mad dog. This is not a cure all. It's nature's own remedy, gathered from the fields and forests. It is composed entirely of roots, gums, leaves, herbs and berries. It purifies the blood, tones up the stomach, quiets the nerves, creates an appetite and brings new life into your system. If you are suffering from that most dreaded of all diseases, rheumatism, take a bottle of my bitters, and if it don't cure you prepare to meet your God, for you've got to die."[63]

Creative jamb pitchmen like Wallace usually expanded their horizons beyond mere street work. Some, like Jim Lighthall, cured by mail as a sideline. Lighthall, an Indian medicine pitchman, included a self-diagnosis sheet in his book, *The Indian Household Medicine Guide,* which was to be torn out

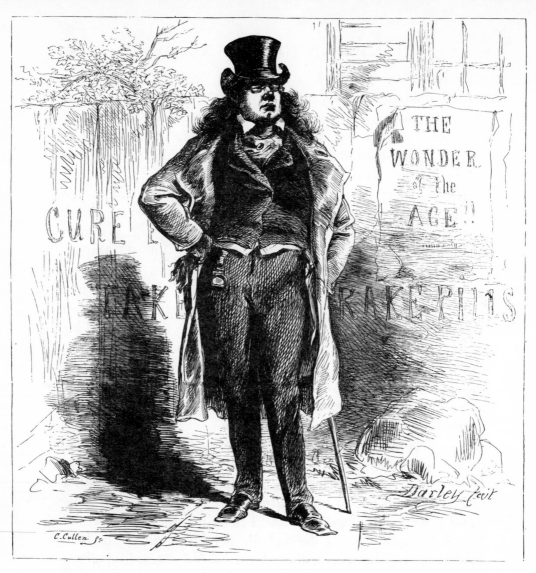

F. O. C. Darley, *The Quack Doctor*, 1871.

and completed by the sufferer and forwarded to the Indian doctor at his "medicine lodge" in Peoria, Illinois. There Lighthall would make a long-distance diagnosis and prescribe the proper remedies from among his store of Indian cure-alls.[64] Other pitchmen set up as traveling physicians or surgeons or carried licensed physicians who performed under their direction.[65]

Country newspapers printed countless warnings against the traveling quack physicians common in rural areas. One editor pleaded with his readers to recognize "that merely because a man comes to town and advertises himself as an eminent surgeon or specialist he is not necessarily a safe man to whom to trust their physical ailments. They should know that a really great specialist is not traveling around little towns doing business in this way. They should know that no really great practitioner would diagnose and treat all diseases such as these people claim to do, without personal continuous contact with the patient. Mark them down as 100% fakers and you won't miss it very far."[66] But the appeal of supposed miracle cures was strong among the ignorant, the superstitious, and those on whom regular physicians had given up hope; and temporary consulting rooms (or case-taking parlors) flourished wherever jamb pitchmen were to be found. For the most part their operators used a street pitch or a medicine show as a blind for the case-taking parlor, which usually drew in far more money than the show.[67]

Although they were sometimes housed in tents, many case-taking parlors consisted of several rooms in a cheap hotel or boardinghouse near the street worker's pitch. The pitchman, said Violet McNeäl, needed to be able to point out the location of his office to the crowd, and to remind them continually that they could obtain free medical consultation and advice only a few steps away.[68] The consultation was handled in a number of ways: often two rooms were used, a reception room staffed by a so-called case taker, and an adjoining office in which the traveling "specialist" held forth.[69] This medical luminary might be the pitchman himself, although often the pitchman posed as the case taker, a kind of combined receptionist and male nurse, using a legitimate doctor in the inner office.[70]

The sort of doctors employed by jamb workers were often too unreliable or too unsteady to be placed in front of audiences: for the most part they were hard luck cases who had lost regular practices because of alcohol, drugs or massive incompetence; but liquor was so often the cause of their decline that any physician connected with a medicine show or a pitch doctor's operation was automatically known to his coworkers as The Boozer.[71] In spite of the difficulties they presented to employers, legitimate doctors were eagerly sought after because of the security offered by their licenses to practice medicine. One showman, shortly after World War I, claimed to be willing to offer physicians a guaranteed weekly salary of one hundred and fifty dollars and 25 percent of a total take that might amount to six or eight hundred dollars a week. He found no difficulty locating interested physicans.[72] Characteristically, the payment was far more modest. "All he wants is a quart of liquor a day," said a pitch doctor about a physician. "Works better with it than without it. Where you're going you can buy good corn for four dollars. Or . . . you could feed him gin at two bucks."[73] Other operators, however, found the doctors more trouble than they were worth. A medicine showman stopped carrying physicians after a single year because he felt their presence irritated local medical men and caused them to be unnecessarily interested in the activities in his consulting room.[74] One of his physicians was especially annoying because of an excess of zeal. Instead of prescribing his employer's tonic for everything from cancer to a head cold, a spark of humanitarianism or a perverse sense of humor led him —to the horror of the showman—to write prescriptions for legitimate drugs and cheerfully send his customers off to the local drugstore to have them filled.[75]

Many case-taking parlors were run by so-called code workers, who substantially improved the odds in diagnosis. When the patient entered the reception room he was told that the doctor was busy. After a few minutes of waiting, the case taker would casually begin a conversation, ultimately drawing out the patient about the details of the ailment that had brought him to the doctor's office. As he talked, the case taker idly toyed with a pencil. A diagnosis card like those sent out by the mail healers was tucked under his left elbow and, as the patient's symptoms came out, they were surreptitiously recorded on the diagnosis card, which was shielded from the patient's view by the case taker's forearm. When he felt that he had enough information, he palmed the card, entered the inner office, ostensibly to see whether the doctor was free, and passed the card to the physician. When the patient entered the doctor's office he was greeted with an astonishing barrage of information about his medical history.[76] "You're talking to a physician now," one code worker told his patients. "Not one of those horse doctors you have around here. I don't have to examine you to tell what's the matter."[77]

Other pitchmen disdained codes, relying solely on their shrewd ability to read the signs of chronic disease and to draw supplementary information from the patient himself without his being aware of it. A medicine man, who ran a case-taking tent in conjunction with his medicine show, told his audiences: "Don't you say where the pain is! You be here tomorrow morning at ten o'clock. You wait your turn; there will be a lot ahead of you. When it's your turn you will be ushered into the little blue tent in the back, that's my office. When you come in there, I want your name, your address, and the kind of work you do. Then I'll do the talking. Don't even say where the misery, the pain, the ache is. We'll tell you.' And we never missed!"[78]

It was vital to the case-taking pitchman that complaints and trouble with the police or local medical societies be kept to a minimum. To protect themselves from legal action, some workers refused to allow a third person in the office when they talked with a patient. "If there are only two of you," said a pitchman named Ed Carlyon, "and if it ever comes to court, your word is as good as his. If there is a third person present, say a friend of the sucker's, he can testify for the sucker. If one of the med bunch is in the room, a smart lawyer might frame a conspiracy charge against you, and that's a felony. Otherwise you're just practicing medicine without a license, and a hundred dollar fine is probably the worst you would get —one or more suckers will make that up fast enough."[79] To avoid trouble Violet McNeal formulated two ironclad rules that governed all her case-taking activities—never to treat a genuinely sick man and never, under any circumstances, to treat a woman, sick or well; women, she believed, were less gullible than men and much more prone to cause trouble if they felt they were victims of a confidence game.[80]

It was the gullibility of the male to which the "medical museums" or "museums of anatomy" owed their existence. The chief purveyors of "manhood" potions, spurious venereal disease cures, and crackpot sexual advice, the medical museums

were set up in red-light districts, near the docks, or in entertainment areas of medium-sized and large cities. The museums
were a combination of the traditional pitchman's case-taking
parlor and the so-called dime museums much favored by
nineteenth- and early twentieth-century tourists. The regular
dime museums created by P. T. Barnum and a host of lesser
showmen were the ancestors of the more recent sideshows or
"ten-in-one's" attached to carnivals and circuses. Generally
they featured a collection of animal, mineral, and vegetable
curiosities, together with human oddities and variety entertainers. Medicine show people often performed in dime museum variety acts, and many of the lecturers who discoursed
on "Baby Alice, the Midget Wonder," the "Dog-Faced Boy,"
and the "Three-Headed Songstress" were veterans of the medicine show platform. It was only natural that medicine showmen would use the museum format to present stationary—if
frequently temporary—medicine shows.[81]

The front windows of most medical museums were designed
to stop the idle passerby in his tracks with some kind of arrest-
ing tableau. The Reinhardt Brothers, owners of a number of
Middle Western museums, made great successes with such
scenes as "The Dying Custer," in which a model of the unfor-
tunate General breathed its last several hundred times each
day thanks to a concealed apparatus inside his tunic. Their
spectacular African jungle scene was described by a St. Paul,
Minnesota, newspaperman: "There were three figures. A white
big-game, pith-helmet type hunter, and two native gun-bearers. Almost at the hunter's feet a huge snake coiled and un-
coiled. The hunter moved forward. The snake struck. The
hunter recoiled, yet did not lose his aplomb, for the pith helmet remained in place. This sequence occupied perhaps one
minute, then the snake coiled again and struck. I remember
that the gun-bearers never moved an inch. They stood with
gaping mouths, fascinated at the drama."[82] The Reinhardts
and their competitors also staged tableaux somewhat more in
their line, generally featuring a cast of automata in one of the
less outrageously grisly medical or surgical scenes. One display, created by the Reinhardts' waxworks foreman, Monsieur
Brouillard, for the Indianapolis museum showed a group on a

Advertisement for a book on "sexual exhaustion."

beach watching a drowning victim being resuscitated by a
man whose arms, like Custer's chest, were activated by some
hidden mechanism. Moving closer to the point, the Reinhardts'
Gary, Indiana, museum featured a window in which a doctor
and nurse tended a syphilitic baby.[83]

As a tourist entered the museum, under a sign reading "For
Men Only," he found himself in a kind of antechamber, usually
nothing more than a corridor lined with glass cases. In the corridor the proprietors displayed wax or papier-mâché models of
the earliest and least loathesome stages of venereal disease,
voluptuous female anatomical models, a few live monkeys,
snakes, or birds, or a miscellaneous collection of curiosities
like those found in most dime museums.[84] About 1870 the New
York Museum of Anatomy featured, among other inducements,
a waxwork, "The Dying Zouave"; a lady's foot which resembled a human face; a man with a horn on his forehead; several
hermaphrodites; "The World-Renowned 'Gertu!' The *Ne Plus
Ultra* of Feminine Beauty"; and a "Galvanic Toilet Bowl."[85]

Once inside the main room, the assault on the patron's
nerves began in earnest. Everywhere about him were glass
cases filled with hideously diseased organs modeled in death-
like wax or luridly painted papier-mâché. The lights were low,
the atmosphere hushed and funereal. Case after case displayed
gaping sores and hideous deformities attributed to syphilis,
gonorrhea, or to that nameless terror of the nineteenth century,
the "secret vice," masturbation. Finally, in the darkest and
most remote corner of the museum, the already shaken tourist
came upon the horror of horrors, an innocuous glass case, totally dark inside. If he paused in front of the case, a light
flashed on and he was confronted with the ghastly visage of a
smirking and drooling idiot boy and the awful legend: "Lost
Manhood." At this point a solicitous "floor man" would appear
from nowhere and begin to talk to the frightened patron. If it
appeared that the customer was in need of medical aid—or
could be convinced that he was—he was steered upstairs to the
"medical institute" run by an "eminent specialist" in the various secret diseases.[86] The so-called medical institute, of course,
was nothing but a version of the ubiquitous case-taking parlor.

Once inside and in the clutches of the "specialist," it was un-

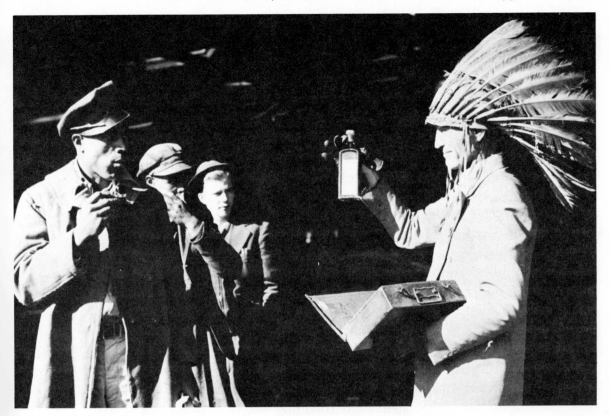

Patent medicine pitchman, Durham, North Carolina, 1939.

LIBRARY OF CONGRESS.

likely that the customer would emerge again until he had spent at least five dollars and often as much as twenty dollars on worthless medication or treatment. For the most part, customers considered the money well spent after hearing a diagnosis of the terrible state of their sex organs. A California physician went through an examination by a "secret diseases" specialist, and left an account of the museum doctor's procedure. After taking a urine sample, the doctor abandoned the sufferer to his fears for an hour or more, finally returning with a long face and announcing in sepulchral tones: "'I don't wish to alarm you, sir, but you are in a bad way. Your urine is full of animalcules. The microscope shows them plainly. Be tranquil, sir; your case is not desperate; but your blood is full of spermatatozoa . . . Now, sir, as long as the animalcules swim endwise there is no difficulty. They circulate all about the body without injury. But let one of them get crosswise, so . . . Don't you see the effect is to obstruct the blood vessel instantly? And then you drop dead, sir!' "[87]

For pitchmen—honest and patently dishonest—the vision of great wealth lay always a bit in the future, with a fresh start in a new territory. Most street workers spent their lives moving restlessly from one place to another, discarding an Indian remedy for an Oriental panacea, always in search of the fantastic drug or unbeatable novelty or fresh approach to selling that would make their fortunes. They purchased copies of *The Spieler, or the Money Maker's Manual,* which promised "novelties, plans, schemes and new systems, strange secrets and new discoveries. The almighty dollar, how to acquire it easily, honorably and quickly."[88] Or they corresponded with Silver Cloud, a dubious Western character who advertised for partners with a thousand dollars, promising "the Biggest, the Newest and Best Proposition on the boards for Store Grind and Office Combined."[89] In their search for the pitchman's pot of gold, many street workers answered the "agents wanted" advertisements placed in the theatrical papers by the patent medicine firms that sponsored traveling shows. Assembling a few musicians, a blackface comedian, and an acrobat or two, they set out on the road as full-fledged medicine showmen.

3

THE MEDICINE SHOW

You are all dying, every man, every woman and child is dying; from the instant you are born you begin to die and the calendar is your executioner. That, no man can change or hope to change. It is nature's law that there is no escape from the individual great finale on the mighty stage of life where each of you are destined to play your farewell performance. Ponder well my words then ask yourselves the questions: Is there a logical course to pursue? Is there some way you can delay, and perhaps for years, that final moment before your name is written down by a bony hand in the cold diary of death? Of course there is, Ladies and Gentlemen, and that is why I am here.

Open Pitch of T. P. Kelley

Medicine shows carrying as few as two or three performers and as many as forty operated throughout the United States and Canada from about 1870 to 1930, and even later in some out of the way areas. The "forty-milers" or "home guard"—often ama-

OREGON INDIAN MEDICINE CO.
BOARD CONTRACT.

Mr_____proprietor of_____Hotel, hereby agrees

to board_____people of Oregon Indian Medicine Co., No._____at the

rate of $_____Dollars per week. All meals lost to be deducted. All extra meals to be

charged for at the same rate. All rooms to be reasonably furnished. Doctors room to have fire; plenty of fuel fur-

nished. Contract to begin with_____ 190 Advance representative to be kept at the same rate.

Signed_____

Dated_____ _____ 190 _____Advance representative.

Room and board contract used by medicine shows representing the
Oregon Indian Medicine Company.

WILLIAM H. HELFAND COLLECTION.

teur medicine men—performed only in the vicinity of their own
towns. In the nineties, for example, Charles T. Hunt, the owner
of a small circus, toured a tiny three-man medicine show for
eleven or twelve weeks each winter in order to get enough
money to take out his circus in the spring. After working up a
week's worth of acts, Hunt, his wife, a comedian, and several
dozen performing dogs took to the road with a line of German
Medicine Company remedies, making the rounds of small halls
near their home in Kingston, New York.[1] The small professional troupes, however, were usually warm weather shows,
staying in their winter quarters until April or May and returning home again in October or November. If the need for money
kept small shows on the road during the winter months, they
headed for the South or played wherever they could find free
or inexpensive shelter, often using schoolhouses, Grange halls,
tobacco barns or vacant stores for their performances.[2] Most
large professional troupes traveled the year round, playing in
halls and small-town opera houses during the winter and in
tents or on open-air stages during the other seasons.[3]

Unlike the pitchman, the medicine showman was essentially
a theatrical producer, packaging shows that were interrupted

HALL OR LOT CONTRACT.

....

Name of Town   State   Date

This Agreement, Made by and between.........................

....

party of the first part and...Manager,

....Hall, party of the second

part, viz: ....

....party of second part agrees to

rent Hall, cleaned, seated, lighted, heated and licensed, known as

...............................Hall, to...to give

entertainments, sell medicine, and conduct their business for a period of

.............consecutive days, commencing on or about ....1 ..

with privilege of as many more days as may be desired for the sum of

.........Dollars for the first week, and.........Dollars for the second week

and each succeeding week, or the proratio for any portion thereof, definite

date of occupancy to be determined by party of first part and party of second

part to be notified accordingly. Party of the second part agrees not to lease

Hall or permit any other Medicine or Electric Belt company to appear in

above place previous to this engagement. In the event of any unforseen

accident or obstacle arising which would make the fulfillment of this cont-

ract impossible, or a three days notice of cancellation by party of first

part, will make this contract null and void, and neither party can be held

responsible for any damage caused thereby .

    Any additions or erasures made in above contract without the approval

of...will in no way be binding upon them.

    Signed, sealed and delivered this.................................day of

.........................A. D. 1   at.................................

                                  ....[SEAL]

                                  ....[SEAL]

If terms of this contract are not satisfactory, please return without erasure.

Stock medicine show hall or lot contract.

periodically for sales pitches and the sales themselves. About one-third of most shows was given over to lectures, demonstrations and sales, and the rest to entertainment, most frequently some sort of variety show.[4] The medicine show operator, as one showman suggested, "had to know everything from booking and advertising to putting up the show and arranging the music."[5] For the operator who could shrewdly balance all of the elements of a medicine show, there was a great deal of money to be made. Before World War I, a number of showmen were making a thousand dollars a week and more after expenses, and many made fortunes on the road which allowed them to retire or go into some other, less controversial form of show business.[6] Percy Williams, for example, piled up a fortune with liver pads which made it possible for him to become an important vaudeville manager, and John Hamlin, one of the originators of the famed Wizard Oil, used his patent medicine millions to become proprietor of the Grand Opera House in Chicago.[7]

Although shows played almost every settled area, the favorite territories were the Middle West and the South. Many companies followed the harvest, playing in the Midwest wheat regions in the summer and moving down toward the cotton towns of the deep South in the fall. Pitchmen and showmen tended to believe that Southerners, especially Southern Negroes, and rural Middle Western types were most easily sold, although some preferred the ethnic audiences found in factory towns in the Middle Atlantic states and New England.[8] T. P. Kelley, a prosperous medicine man, insisted that Ohio was the state most frequented by showmen between 1880 and 1920, with strong competition coming from Michigan, Wisconsin, Illinois, and Indiana.[9] The state treated Kelley well. "I have made more money in small Ohio villages," he said, "than I did in fair-size towns in other states, and when playing around Akron, Youngstown, Springfield, and Columbus, where I could be pulling in crowds of six to eight thousand, on blow-off nights when the natives would raise their hands, holding bills and eager to buy my remedies, from the stage platform it would appear like a waving sea of currency was before me. It was a beautiful sight."[10] Harry Leon Wilson's character,

Sooner Jackson, chose Iowa as the medicine man's paradise. "Iowa," he said, "skins pretty . . . three hundred and sixty-five days in the year and in leap year one day more. In fact, give me Iowa, where the boobs . . . simply come up and ask to be had . . . and I wouldn't crave another state out of our whole glorious union. A guy . . . with any savvy . . . needn't ever step across its border. They tell me that in some places out on the edge they still buy lightning-rods and almost everyone you meet will be wearing the Little Wonder Electric Tibetan rheumatism ring. I know because I sold them."[11]

The largest troupes often played fair-sized towns and cities, usually setting up on a circus lot or wherever there was vacant space for their tents in working-class neighborhoods. Smaller companies played little towns and villages for the most part, relying on the fact that country people would frequently travel great distances on the expectation of seeing a medicine show and perhaps of being cured of an ailment from which they had been suffering for some time.[12] Flo St. John, who ran small shows with her husband, estimated that country people, starved for entertainment, made up 90 percent of her audiences.[13] Anna Mae Noell, whose parents operated a small outfit called the Jack Roach Indian Medicine Show, talked of playing towns "too small for real theatre, nickelodeons or Chautauqua." "It was long before radio and TV," she added, "and this was the only kind of entertainment the yokels ever got to see. They loved it, and out of gratitude they bought whatever my father and mother sold them."[14] Milton Bartok found country people an eager and profitable audience into the forties and even the fifties: "The Bartok show was a gathering place in each town. They had no TV, and they used to come to the lot well before each show. There would be visiting on a large scale, like at a country church. Some people would meet relatives from two towns away that they hadn't talked to in a couple of years. When the tent was up and ready to go we would send our band down on a truck with banners on it saying, 'Free Show. Big Free Show. Bartok Medicine Company. Bardex, the World's Medicine.' The first night we would have a fair crowd; the next night that crowd should double."[15]

In comparison to the pitchman, who needed nothing more

than his tripes and keister, his pan torches, and perhaps a suit-case filled with spare clothing, even a small medicine show carried a fair amount of equipment. And the process of moving it from one town to another, especially in wet weather, was often a nightmare filled with mud, injuries to horses and drivers, and damaged equipment. (When Paul Dresser, the song writer, was traveling with a medicine show company during bad weather his wagon supposedly slid down a steep grade outside West Terre Haute, Indiana, and fell into the river, drowning all the performers but Dresser.[16]) It was to the showman's benefit to stay in one place as long as possible, especially in bad weather, and operators tried to remain in small towns at least a week and preferably two.[17] Large important companies that could draw huge crowds would work cities for as long as two months at a time.[18]

Although an advance agent scouted territories for many shows, and others worked the same general circuits for years at a time, it was not always possible for showmen to tell the good towns from the bad. In order to be prepared for a possible string of bad towns, medicine men were careful—especially before the widespread use of trucks gave them genuine mobility—never to play into a territory that they could not play out of by another route in case of emergency. A good town might acquire a hostile sheriff or experience a city hall shake-up that removed vital people from power. Some towns, of course, were perennially anti-medicine show and charged prohibitive license fees or merely made certain that there was never a place to perform. Others, like Ingersoll, Ontario, known as the "Graveyard of medicine show men," were simply towns that did not buy medicine for whatever mysterious reasons.[19] All of Canada, in fact, presented fairly considerable sales resistance. A Canadian medicine wholesaler informed an American medicine man that not only were laws very strict regarding medicine, and the license fees high, but that "Canada is not the U.S.A., and the people are very cautious in buying."[20]

Most troupes moved by wagon, only gradually switching to trucks after the turn of the century, with company members either boarding at nearby hotels, living in tents, or in later years following the caravan in their own house cars or trailers.[21] A

few large companies traveled by rail, performing on a circus
lot next to a railroad siding or hiring local vans to "gilly" their
shows from the siding to their lot or hall and back again.[22]
The Great Mac Ian's Mastodon Medicine Company and Oliver
Cornet Band and Orchestra traveled from place to place in
style in the private car of Dr. Ian Mack, the proprietor. "The
car," a news item recounted, "has been remodeled and re-
painted and christened Lil-gar. The entire company stops at
hotels, as the car is used by the doctor for his private use, while
an engagement is being played."[23] It was not always easy to
find hotels for medicine show people. The reputation of all performers was notoriously low with keepers of hotels and board-
inghouses, expecially in rural areas, and medicine show people
were considered by many to be especially unreliable. Some
shows booked accommodations ahead through an advance
agent who had a way with hotel clerks and suspicious land-
ladies. The Oregon Indian Medicine Company supplied free
packets of board contracts to troupes handling their products.
The contracts grandly informed the wary innkeeper that "The
entertainments given by the Oregon Indian Medicine Co. are
not to be confounded or classified with any other so-called Indian Medicine Company. Their reputation and responsibilities
are too great. This is One of Our Best Shows Under a Model
Manager. WE TEACH VIRTUE, MORALITY, AND HEALTH."[24]

Most companies booked their halls and lots using stock
questionnaires and contract forms ordered from job printers or
supplied free to showmen by patent medicine wholesalers.[25] A
typical questionnaire, used by the East Indian Remedy Company, was sent out to managers of public halls and opera
houses with a stamped return envelope some weeks in advance
of a potential tour. Under a letterhead advertising East Indian
Remedies was a cautious message to managers followed by a
form to be filled out and returned to the main office of the company:

Dear Sir:—
   We intend to visit your town in the near future and
ask you to fill out the following questions and return
to the address below.

Manager of Public, or Opera Hall.

————

. . . . .190. .

Dear Sir,—

        Please fill out the Blanks in regards to the following questions and oblige us. As we intend visiting your town at an early date, you will confer an extreme favor upon me by returning thes as soon as possible in enclosed stamped envelope.

Yours very truly.

———

Name of Town . . . . Population . . . .

Has a Medicine Company been in your town . . . .

If so how long ago? . . . . Name of Opera Hall Mgr. . . . .

Is Opera Hall Licensed, ... Have you Stage aud Scenery, ...

Very Lowest Price per week . . . . How many Seats . . . .

Name number of Factories in your town . . . .

Have you the Weeks of . . . . open, ...

If not, what are the first open weeks, ...

GIVE VERY LOWEST RENT IN FIRST LETTER.

Stock questionnaire sent to managers of halls and theatres by medicine shows.

> We carry a nice company with us, consisting of la-
> dies and gentlemen, and leave only the best reputa-
> tion in each town we visit. We come to your town for
> the purpose of advertising Our Own Celebrated Rem-
> edies and will be pleased to hear from you as soon as
> possible, as we are now booking ahead.

Managers were advised to answer the following questions
without fail since their responses went on file and would be
used again by the company:

> What is the name of your House? Where located? Is it
> well lighted and seated? What kind of light? How
> many seats? What kind? How big is the house? What
> floor is it located on? Have you piano or organ? Have
> you stage curtain and scenery? Is your house li-
> censed? Has there been a company of our nature
> there before? When? What was the name of it? State
> your lowest price per week, lighted, heated, cleaned,
> with use of piano, or organ, etc. Or will you play us
> on percentage? If so, what percent? Name and num-
> ber of factories in your town? Have you weeks of
> _____ open? If not, what are your first open weeks?
> What is correct population of your village? Not the
> township. How many halls in your town? By whom
> owned? Have you a hotel in village? Give name.[26]

If the terms stated in the returned questionaire seemed satisfactory, a completed contract was returned to the manager
for his signature by an advance agent or by mail. A standard
contract form called for the management to make certain that
the premises were "cleaned, seated, lighted, heated and licensed," and that the space had not been recently leased to
"any other Medicine or Electric Belt company."[27] The contract
was handily cancelable "in the event of any unforeseen accident or obstacle arising which would make the fulfillment of
this contract impossible, or a three days notice of cancellation" by the showman.

The characteristic local opera house had probably never
been host to a genuine operatic performance. The term had

arisen and become popular, especially in the Midwest and the West, because the word "theatre" was in distinctly ill repute during much of the nineteenth century.[28] Every progressive hamlet, however, yearned for an opera house to supplement the facilities offered by town halls and lodge rooms. Many opera houses were built by local magnates with a cosmopolitan bent or those whose wives and daughters possessed cultural aspirations. Others were erected by local subscription or financed by city governments. Their common fare was an awesomely respectable round of strawberry festivals, temperance lectures, graduation exercises, and church fairs, tempered by occasional performances of traveling repertory companies, minstrel shows, and the offerings of the medicine showmen.

In good weather, showmen used lots in preference to halls because of the smaller expense involved in playing outside and, in the case of big shows drawing very large crowds, because of the need for a generous amount of space. Some showmen refused to play halls because they would not hold sufficient audience to make it worth their while, a not unreasonable consideration in an era when important companies claimed to draw crowds of five or six thousand in a single night.[29] For ordinary companies, however, the audience might number no more than a few dozen or at best far short of a thousand, and small-town opera houses were welcome since they substantially extended the usual outdoor playing season.

Medicine shows that worked outdoors generally played from the back of a specially equipped wagon or later a housecar, from a platform, or inside a tent of some kind. The smallest shows almost invariably worked without a tent, and many carried no seats, forcing spectators to stand or sit on the ground during the performance. Dr. Hill traveled in an elaborate wagon not unlike a gypsy's caravan, with a small stage at the back around which the audience gathered. The central attraction of Hill's peculiar wagon-stage was a crane or boom that was cantilevered from the back of the wagon. At the beginning of the performance the boom telescoped out over the audience carrying Hill's pretty young wife, who did a dance above the heads of the spectators. To discourage undue familiarity, Hill wired his wife to an electric coil which delivered a massive

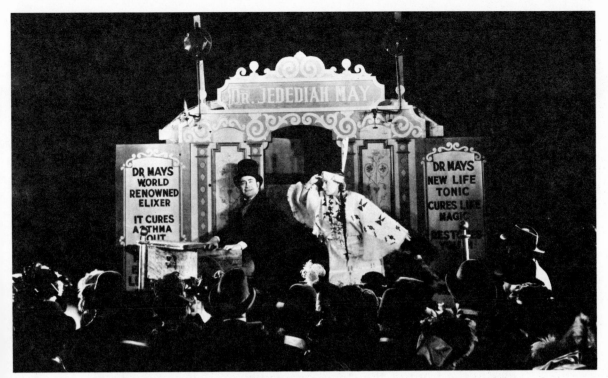

Reconstruction of a medicine show wagon stage from *Swing High*, with Helen Twelvetrees, Pathé, 1930.

PICTURE COLLECTION, NEW YORK PUBLIC LIBRARY.

Reconstruction of a medicine show stage from *The Kid Brother*, with Harold Lloyd, Paramount, 1927.

PICTURE COLLECTION, NEW YORK PUBLIC LIBRARY.

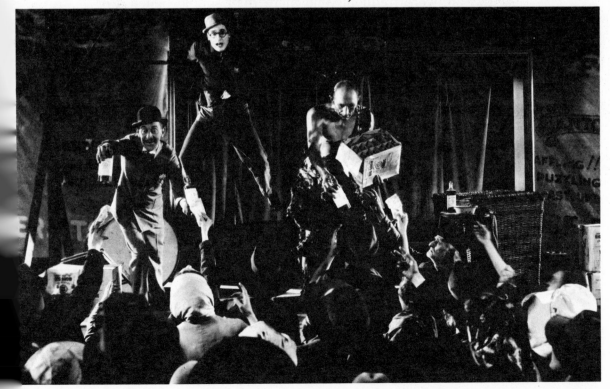

shock to anyone on the ground unwise enough to reach up for a pat or pinch.[30]

The majority of medicine shows operated from simple free-standing stages that resembled the traditional mountebank's booth. Most consisted of little more than a raised platform with a wooden upright at each corner supporting the frame for a striped awning canvas top. The rear and, in some cases, the sides of the stage were also enclosed with canvas, and the front occasionally boasted a curtain suspended from rings on a wire stretched between the uprights. T. P. Kelley's outdoor stage was a typical "five-foot high and eighteen-foot square medicine show platform with slender cross-beams rising above it. A brown canvas backdrop at the rear of the stage, the wooden steps behind that led up to it and side-wings for entrance and exit."[31] Many shows also used an additional smaller platform, essentially a runway jutting out into the audience at right angles to the front of the stage, for medicine pitches and sales.[32] Until the twenties, when electric lights became more common, most outdoor shows illuminated their stages with the typical pitchman's gasoline or kerosene pan torches, although troupes that could afford it sometimes mounted a calcium floodlight on a pole at the rear of the audience area. Seats, when they were used at all, were frequently no more than simple benches or planks laid across soapboxes. The area that contained the stage and the spectators was sometimes enclosed with a rope barrier or a roofless sidewall tent, and a barker's stand like those used in front of circus side shows was occasionally set up just outside the entrance, where the acts could give a sample of their work and the lecturer expound before the show.[33]

Roofless tents (sometimes called airodrome tents) were popular with showmen because they were cheaper, easier to carry, and far less difficult to set up and strike than a conventional circus top. One showman speculated that their popularity also arose in part because audiences always began to worry that a conventional roofed tent would blow down on them as soon as the least gust of wind appeared, and that such anxiety interfered seriously with medicine sales.[34] The prospect of an anxious audience, however, did not deter showmen who could afford it from buying roofed tents, which made it possible for them to perform even in fairly wet or chilly weather. The Big Sensation Medicine Company seated 1,500 spectators in a sixty-foot round top with a sixty-foot middle piece, forming a "canvas theatre 60 by 120 feet, with some 40 feet at one end for an ornately draped stage, carried off at each side with masking curtains, and back of [which] were the dressing rooms, partitioned off to make two on a side."[35] In front of the stage were five hundred folding chairs, and rising behind them bleachers for one thousand more sufferers. Around such shows would be a welter of other tents, housing cooking and dining facilities for performers, offices, consulting rooms, and temporary stockpiles of the medicine being sold.[36]

Many medicine shows had no admission charge, although some charged from two cents up to fifteen or twenty, especially on Wednesday nights when a "double show" with shortened lectures and more entertainment meant reduced medicine sales.[37] The admission charge was not expected to pay for the show in any case, and one showman claimed that he would gladly have paid audiences ten cents a head to be exposed to his lectures.[38] Small shows depended chiefly on the immediate sale of medicine and the prize candy which virtually every troupe carried; larger shows, which generally handled their own brands, made money on drugstore sales after the departure of the troupe. Milton Bartok told his audiences: " 'We got medicine, yeah. If you want to buy the medicine, you buy it. If you don't want to buy it, you don't have to. Nobody makes you buy it. You want to buy it at the drug store? I'd rather you buy it at the drug store. You know the few bottles we sell here don't pay for this show. But I know the medicine's so good that when we leave here you're going to buy it ten years from now.' And they did."[39]

A surprisingly large amount of money was made from the prize candy that was a fixture of most medicine shows. Troupes that drew big audiences could take in several hundred dollars from candy at a single show, and some actually made more money from candy sales than from medicine.[40] The lure was not so much the candy itself but the prizes that were offered to those who bought it. The candy arrived in two cartons from one of the companies that specialized in supplying shows, usually pricing their merchandise so that showmen were virtually guaranteed a hundred percent profit.[41] In the first carton was the candy—small boxes that contained some cheap confection and either a tiny prize or a prize slip that entitled the possessor to claim a more substantial reward from the stage. The second box contained the prize slip items—often quilts, blankets or bedspreads because they were relatively inexpensive and because a few served as impressive "flash" at the rear of the stage.[42] During the show, perhaps four major prizes would be given away, including such items as French dolls, dish sets, pot and pan sets, watches, and giant pandas, and perhaps one smaller prize (a vanity lamp, a pillow or a cut-glass bowl reminiscent of the "slum" given out at carnival booths) for every ten boxes of candy sold.[43] At one show, spectators received joke books, manicure sets, napkin rings, cigarette holders, scissors, goggles, pocket knives, and whistles.[44] Often, because the candy was inexpensive, it would be sold as the first item of the evening to start the money flowing. Some showmen, however, preferred to start with a cheap medicine or soap and finish the evening with the candy sale and distribution of prizes.[45]

For the most part, medicine shows handled the same remedies and medical appliances as the pitchmen, although the shows did not ordinarily deal in the nonmedical novelties sold by street workers. The staples of the medicine show generally included an herb compound with some tonic or cathartic properties, a liniment or oil, a salve, a catarrh cure, a corn remedy, and some sort of medicated soap. Like the pitchman, medicine show owners prepared their own cures or ordered them from patent medicine manufacturers, who generally bottled the showman's own formula or merely pasted his personal label on their own stock liniment or herb remedy.

A number of the preparations sold by medicine shows were manufactured in hotel bathtubs or in washtubs hauled out from under the show platform when a new batch of tonic was required. Ingredients were bought from the local drugstore as needed or from chemical wholesalers.[46] Violet McNeal streamlined the process by keeping her private formula on file with a large drug house that would send out the premixed medicines in 110-pound drums. She would bottle and label the compound herself as it was needed.[47] A "snake oil" showman bought his product from a Canadian manufacturer already bottled for twenty-five dollars a gross. He had the labels printed locally and advertised the concoction as genuine snake oil, good for arthritis, rheumatism, and similar disorders. Because he had no idea what the bottle contained beyond the fact that it was certainly not snake oil, the showman had the printer add a skull and crossbones and an ominous warning that the concoction was not to be taken internally.[48] Other showmen bought a prelabeled mixture with their own name printed in as manufacturer.[49] The great majority, however, usually handled some standard brand ordered from a wholesale druggist or from one of the patent medicine manufacturers: the sarsaparillas of the Ayer and Hood companies were popular, along with such perennials as Merchant's Gargling Oil, Wright's Indian Vegetable Pills, and Lydia E. Pinkham's Vegetable Compound.

The laboratories that supplied showmen existed in bewildering variety.[50] One supplier, Dr. R. B. Webb, housed his laboratory in a tiny unpainted shack. A crudely lettered sign over the door informed customers that they were entering DR. WEBB'S LAB. MFG. OF INDIAN HERB MEDICINE. CURES WHEN OTHERS FAIL. TRY OUR SPECIAL RED-DEVIL SALVES FOR OLD CARONIC [sic] SORES. IND. BLOOD TONIC BUILDS UP LOST MAN-HOOD.[51] There were dozens of more reliable suppliers, catering exclusively or in large part to medicine shows. A typical small operation was the Clifton Remedy Company of Girard, Illinois, founded in 1899 by Abraham Lincoln Dix and Dr. Henry W. Clifton.[52] The company was established when Clifton, who was running a medicine show in Springfield, was arrested for operating without a license. Dix heard about Clifton's difficulties while in a Springfield gambling house, bailed out the showman, and the two became partners in a patent medicine wholesale operation, which grossed $35,000 in its best year, 1926, and finally ceased to operate in 1954.

The Clifton Remedy Company made thirteen products, including headache tablets, catarrh snuff, corn salves, healing salves, liniments, and laxatives. The herbs and raw drugs used in the preparation of their products came from a drug house in Peoria, their bottles from Alton, and the cartons from Chicago.

At the peak of their production, during the twenties, the com-pany had eight regular employees who mixed headache pow-ders and concocted the salves and liniments. The pills were rolled by larger pharmaceutical manufacturers. The Clifton Company sold both to drug wholesale houses which supplied medicine showmen and, through advertisements in *The Bill-board,* directly to the showmen themselves. As many as forty shows at a time bought the Clifton products, usually ordering once a week by mail. The direct sales to medicine men were made virtually at cost, the company's chief profit coming from repeat orders from drugstores in the towns where medicine shows had played. During the twenties, for example, the retail price of the Clifton laxative was $12.00 a dozen. Druggists pur-chased it for $8.00 a dozen and wholesalers for 15 percent less; but medicine showmen were able to buy the same mixture direct for $1.15 a dozen because, in effect, their shows were ad-vertising the preparation for the Clifton Remedy Company.

One of the largest suppliers of patent medicines to showmen was Frank P. Horne's German Medicine Company of Cincin-nati. The tradition of the High German Doctor, from which Horne drew his inspiration, was an ancient one, extending back to the mountebanks of the Renaissance. Probably because of the high regard in which German universities were held, quacks with foreign accents and a penchant for spouting scientific jar-gon often passed themselves off as German or German-edu-cated physicians. "I am the High-German Doctor," announced one mountebank, "who, by the blessing of Aesculapius on his great Pains, Travels and Nocturnal Lucubrations, has attained to a greater share of knowledge than any person before him was ever known to do."[53] The drugs dispensed by High Ger-man Doctors were believed to be the products of great skill and learning, and so-called German remedies like Hoofland's German Tonic and Schiffmann's German Asthma Cure re-mained popular in America until World War I sent proprietors in search of less controversial origins for their tonics.

The German Medicine Company was an extensive operation, often supplying a hundred shows at a time with Teutonia, Germania Oil, the Berlin Corn and Bunion Cure, and several dozen other preparations.[54] To expedite telegraph orders from

TO-NIGHT!

GERMAN MEDICINE CO.

The Popular
LADY CONTEST
Will Be Decided
TO=NIGHT.

**The Lucky Contestant will receive a
Handsome Present.**

Big Bill, Special Features,
TO=NIGHT.

Stock dodger, German Medicine Company.

showmen, the company worked out a code system which they explained in a brochure directed to medicine men. The code allowed one to send most messages for ten words or less, cut down errors, and, it was stressed, made secrecy possible—unless, of course, a rival had received the same brochure.[55] Basically, the code worked like the charts for determining the distance between two cities found on road maps. Down one side of the chart was a list of all the German remedies; across the top was a series of columns representing quantities, from one bottle or box up to five gross. The showmen found the key word at a point of intersection; an order of nine dozen small bottles of Germania Oil, for example, was represented by the code word "Cane." Additional words were supplied at the bottom of the chart. A sample message supplied by the company was: "Variety tumble open cactus nabob unco babe jet powder eureka." The decoded message read: "Send by fast freight, 6 doz. Teutonia 3 doz. Germania Oil 1 doz. Horne's cough syrup ¼ doz. Queen of the Valley 1 Gross Berlin corn cure 1 doz. Puri-Fi-Curi soap assorted paper, send me an A.1. all around performer that plays organ."[56]

In addition to supplying their own brands, the German Medicine Company was willing to undertake preparation of medicines under any showman's personal label.[57] But the value of the free advertising provided by showmen who carried German Medicine Company products was not lost on the proprietor, who urged medicine men to sell the German line rather than a personal brand and offered the inducement of free promotional materials to those who did. "The advantage of handling the German Remedies is the elegant assortment of advertising novelties, paper etc. which we furnish FREE, all you can use of it. Paper will be sent to you for the asking."[58] To medicine showmen, free "paper" (posters, flyers, trade cards, tickets, and the like) was an important incentive because it saved substantially on printers' bills and helped to give the impression that an independent troupe was actually an advertising unit of one of the well-known patent medicine firms when in fact the troupe did nothing more than sell the products of the company. Since large patent medicine firms could order standardized posters and throwaways in huge lots for pennies, and since it was to their benefit to have their name advertised even by second-rate troupes because of the important repeat drugstore sale, companies like Horne's distributed paper with a lavish hand.

The large colored advertising poster was popularized by the circus and the Wild West show. By the nineties it had been adopted by a wide variety of business enterprises, and walls and fences everywhere were plastered with elaborate and brightly colored advertisements for theatres, patent medicines, soap, and tobacco.[59] The staple of poster advertising was the one-sheet, which was twenty-eight by forty-two inches in size. With this as base, advertisers employed one-half-, two-, three- and four-sheets, each of which was printed on a single piece of paper. A six-sheet, for example, was made up of two three-sheets; and eight-, sixteen-, and twenty-four-sheets were made from four-sheet posters.[60] The smaller posters, up to the four-sheet size, were frequently used in store windows, while larger posters were placed on board fences or the sides of barns, where they generally remained until pulled down or covered by bill posters working for a rival company.[61] For the cost of the freight, the German Medicine Company supplied its customers with packages containing twenty-two posters, ranging in size from one-eighth sheet to twenty-sheet.[62] Along with the posters came packets of smaller paper items, including cheap promotional magazines like those given out by some circuses and Wild West shows, pamphlets on German products, trade cards, circulars, and throwaways or "dodgers" advertising the German Medicine Company's "HIGH CLASS Vaudeville," with "Sterling Specialties, Dainty Dancers, Clever Comedians, Sweet Singers" in "An unrivalled array of bright and catchy AMUSEMENT."[63] Depending upon the version of the dodger used by the showman, admission to this "CONTINUOUS ROUND OF PLEASURE" was two cents, five cents, ten cents, twenty cents, or gratis.[64] Also available were admission tickets, present tickets, most beautiful baby votes, bean guesses, most popular lady votes, contracts, route sheets, stationery, picture postcards, rulers, mirrors, codes and other novelties.[65]

The obvious—and intentional—impression given to the public was that any troupe using German Medicine Company paper was an official advertising unit of the company. Most large suppliers followed suit. In fact, relatively few patent medicine houses actually sent out sponsored troupes because of the expense and the management problems involved. But two of those that did—the Hamlin Company and the Kickapoo Indian Medicine Company—produced the best known and the most popular American medicine shows.

4

WIZARD OIL

Oh! I love to travel far and near throughout my native land;
I love to sell as I go 'long, and take the cash in hand.
I love to cure all in distress that happen in my way,
And you better believe I feel quite fine when folks rush up and say:

CHORUS:
"I'll take another bottle of Wizard Oil,
I'll take another bottle or two;
I'll take another bottle of Wizard Oil,
I'll take another bottle or two."

Carl Sandburg,
The American Songbag

Before the turn of the nineteenth century there had developed all sorts of exotic approaches to medicine show business, guaranteed—at least in theory—to stun the locals into parting with their cash. Among them was the Indian medicine show, essentially a scaled-down version of the Wild West show with a heavy dose of vaudeville and blackface minstrelsy thrown in for good measure, and the Oriental shows, madly eclectic entertainments aimed at tantalizing what one showman termed the "whistlers, whittlers, and spitters" of the farm country.[1] Sometimes the two forms merged in especially bizarre combinations. One Indian troupe featured Elita, a mind reader who informed audiences that she had been born with a veil over her face, and that she was the thirteenth daughter of an Arabian mother, born on the thirteenth day of the month, who could trace her ancestors to the thirteenth century.[2] And a

Kickapoo Indian Medicine Company unit, in a burst of internationalism, hired a Hindu, Dr. Punja, to lecture on American Indian remedies.[3] Nevada Ned's Hindoo Patalka show featured Oliver himself, sporting an elaborate buckskin frontier outfit, two Syrians hired out of a rug store, a Hindu who had been doing a vaudeville magic act, and a borrowed elephant which ended the tour by crashing through the floor of a bridge in New Jersey.[4]

Such eccentricity and light-mindedness did not always go unnoticed. In New England and Bible Belt communities, especially, there was a long tradition of hostility to all sorts of performers. Some liberal spirits in such places defended traveling shows as rational and instructive amusement, but to many rural people, well into the twentieth century, any form of theatre represented the broad road to destruction. This disdain for the theatrical, coupled with a time-honored distrust of the mountebank, forced medicine showmen to defend the morality of their performers and the educational value of their shows and lectures to hostile critics. In their advertising and on the lecture platform, medicine showmen trumpeted their performances as strictly moral and educational family entertainment. "We come in here, bring you nice free show," Marton Bartok told his audiences. "Anything wrong with the show? Anything bad? Anything that the priest, the preacher, your children shouldn't hear? No!"[5] Some went a step further than mere talk and attempted to manufacture credibility by giving their shows a quasi-religious tone.

The proprietors of the Quaker shows, for example, usually appeared on the platform in characteristic fawn-colored Quaker dress, with wide-brimmed, low-crowned hats and "barn-door" trousers that buttoned up the sides. They larded their lectures with "thee" and "thou" and "Brother," and solemnly blessed the customers at the end of each medicine sale.[6] The Quaker Doctors or Healers, of course, had absolutely no connection with the Religious Society of Friends, but merely a strong interest in trading on the Quaker reputation for honesty and fair dealing. Once the initial piety was over, however, their shows generally became something less than Quakerish. One so-called "Quaker Doctor and Optician," for example, who performed at the Opera House in West Bend, Indiana, advertis-

HAMLIN'S
WIZARD OIL

THE GREAT MEDICAL WONDER.

There is no Sore it will Not Heal, No Pain it will not Subdue.

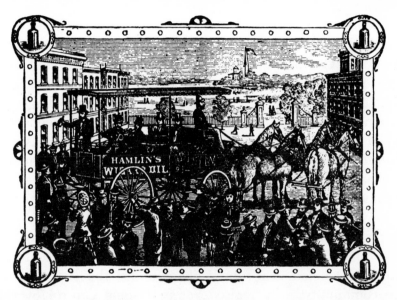

HAMLIN'S COUGH BALSAM

PLEASANT TO TAKE
MAGICAL IN ITS EFFECTS.

HAMLIN'S
BLOOD AND LIVER PILLS
For Liver Complaint, Constipation,
AND ALL
Disorders of the Stomach and Digestive Organs.

PREPARED AT THE LABORATORY 01
HAMLINS WIZARD OIL COMPANY, CHICAGO, ILL.

ing a company of twelve entertainers, "illustrated songs," and a moving picture show.[7] Beason, a celebrated Quaker Doctor, featured a spectacular Negro quartette: "the men with bulldog yellow shoes, three inch white collars and wide-brimmed fedoras, the women with leg-o'-mutton sleeves, wasp waists, high buttoned shoes and peek-a-boo hats."[8] Brother John, dressed in his drab Quaker clothing, would gallop through the crowd awaiting his appearance in a huge chariot drawn by rearing horses.[9]

A somewhat more consistent note of piety was struck by the so-called Shaker troupes sent out by Dr. Lou Turner's Shaker Medicine Company.[10] Turner's company, which had headquarters in St. Louis, Missouri, operated under a special arrangement with the Shaker community of Union Village, near Lebanon, Ohio. In 1833 a botanical garden had been established at Union Village by Abiathar Babbitt and Andrew Houston, two Shaker physicians who served the community and nearby towns. It was from this garden that Turner later obtained the plants and herbs used in Turner's Consumption Cure, or Shaker Cough Remedy; Doctor Turner's Wonder Herbs, the Great Shaker Blood Cure; and Turner's New Life for Women. The remedies, for the most part, were actually bottled and labeled at Union Village under the supervision of the community, which also exercised some control over the way in which Turner marketed their products.[11] Members of his advertising units were prohibited from impersonating Shakers, wearing the characteristic clothing of the sect, or presenting entertainments that would reflect unfavorably on the Shakers. Turner abided by the rules, carrying nothing but companies of psalm singers, and preserving a shatteringly high moral tone. It was only when he discovered that psalm singing was a theatrical fiasco that he added mild conventional shows and lecturers in traditional Shaker garb.[12]

The Wizard Oil Company represented the acme of piety and rectitude. The company, which operated out of Chicago, was founded in the seventies by John Hamlin, a former traveling magician, and his brother Lysander.[13] Wizard Oil, as the Hamlins promoted it, was a liniment with a difference; not only could it be used for common rheumatic pains and sore muscles, it was advertised as a sovereign cure for a whole list of other

Sixteen-sheet Wizard Oil poster.

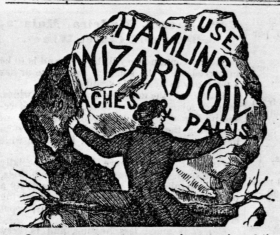

Wizard Oil advertisement.   CHICAGO HISTORICAL SOCIETY.

afflictions, including pneumonia, cancer, and hydrophobia.[14] In fact, Wizard Oil was a respectable but scarcely wonderworking liniment, containing camphor, ammonia, chloroform, sassafras, cloves, and turpentine—and at various times from 55 to 70 percent alcohol, which made it a hair-raising tipple when taken internally, as it was for a number of ailments.[15] Unlike most medicine troupes, the companies sent out by the Hamlins from their Chicago headquarters were genuine advertising units, the chief function of which was to stock druggists with a blood and liver pill, a cough remedy, and the famous liniment, at the same time creating a demand for the Hamlin products with musical performances. Only Wizard Oil, in fifty-cent and dollar bottles, was generally sold to spectators at their famous musical entertainments.[16]

Although the Hamlins experimented with performances in

local halls and opera houses, they concentrated on open-air shows, often extending their seasons by moving far south during the winter months. A Hamlin unit traveled in a special wagon with a surrey top and advertisements for Wizard Oil emblazoned in gigantic letters across the sides. Drawn by four- or six-horse teams, each wagon was in fact a small rolling stage with a built-in parlor organ and lockers under the seats for a week's worth of medicine. Because of the limited space, members of the unit were allowed only hand luggage, which was strapped to the wagon's top; their trunks were shipped ahead to each weekend stop.[17]

The composition of the unit was always the same—a driver, a lecturer, and a vocal quartet that doubled in brass. Their shows combined the usual medicine lecture and sale with vocal and instrumental music and community singing. Like Kickapoo and other large companies that sold medicine on the road, the Hamlin units presented spectators with a version of the traditional patent medicine almanac—in this case the famous "songsters." The songsters, which appeared under such titles as *Hamlin's Wizard Oil New Book of Songs,* and *The Book of Songs As Sung by the Wizard Oil Concert Troupes,* were also available from druggists, and for a one-cent stamp from the main office of the Wizard Oil Company.[18] Typically, they contained several dozen paragraphs of pseudomedical advice on various illnesses, all of which could be cured by Hamlin products, and the lyrics of fifteen or twenty songs, generally such innocuous sentimental or comic pieces as "The Old Red Cradle," "Listen to My Tale of Woe," "The Agricultural Irish Girl," and "Grandfather's Old Brown Pants."[19]

The whole tone of the Hamlin shows was conservative and rigidly proper. There were certain lapses, of course, such as the use of a standard medicine show deafness demonstration in which the ears of a deaf volunteer were briskly rubbed with Wizard Oil and then "popped" by the medicine man, causing a dramatic but temporary restoration of hearing in many cases.[20] But on the whole the Hamlin units were models of exaggerated decorum—"the last word in class, dignity and social distinction."[21] William Burt, a member of a quartet called The Lyceum Four, traveled with a typically correct Hamlin unit be-

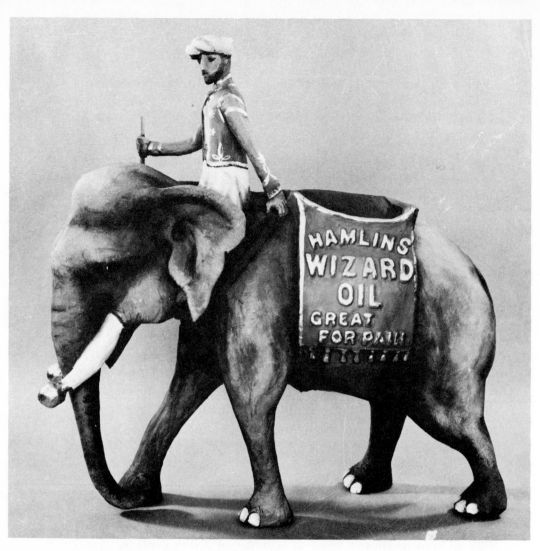

Papier-mâché drugstore display piece. CHICAGO HISTORICAL SOCIETY.

fore the turn of the century. "We appeared," Burt said, "in frock coats, then called 'Prince Alberts,' with the customary gray dress vests and pin-striped trousers, topped off with high silk hats and . . . pearl-gray spats over patent leather shoes. The trousers might be changed for a pair with a wider stripe and the vest could be buff or white linen, with fawn spats exchanged for the pearl-gray, but when one decided to make the changes, so did we all. It was a hard and fast rule, and in order to avoid confusion, we scheduled our weekly changes. This uniform style of dressing was a trademark of all Wizard Oil advertising units. . . . The most vivid recollection of this engagement was a two dollar fine—arbitrarily deducted from my salary—for daring to enter a public dining room wearing a roll collar. Wing collars were the only style for the well-dressed Wizard Oil entertainer regardless of time or place."[22]

To reinforce the already high moral tone of the Hamlin operations, troupe managers volunteered the services of their performers for church fairs and charity bazaars, and every Sunday saw the Wizard Oil singers augmenting the efforts of some local church choir.[23] Because of their good reputation, Wizard Oil companies were able to remain in the same town for as long as six weeks at a time, usually acting with the blessing if not the outright sponsorship of important local institutions.[24] The situation was a tempting one for cheap imitators, and many companies peddling "Wizard Oil" or "Magic Oil" or "Lightning Oil" appeared and traded on the Hamlin reputation for honesty and uplifting entertainment.[25]

A so-called Wizard Oil Company, run by a character who claimed to be Hamlin himself, played towns in the Middle West in the eighties. Although his troupe peddléd Wizard Oil and dispensed songsters to the crowd, the show itself was not the characteristic concert format, but a standard two-man variety bill with Dutch, Irish, and Negro comedy, organ music, two-character comedy sketches, and magic.[26] The Hamlin Company, which rigidly discouraged innovation among its road units, had certainly never heard of this particular operation, which probably forged labels and bought songsters in large numbers from druggists stocked by the genuine Hamlin troupes.[27]

William Burt, after leaving the Hamlin unit, toured for a time with a cheap imitator of the Wizard Oil format, a physician who had taken to the road after a nervous breakdown.[28] The doctor pushed his liniment as a rheumatism cure, and like many other rheumatism specialists, had developed an effective stage presentation in which a combination of persuasive talk and vigorous massage caused some cripples to be able to throw away their crutches and walk a few steps. The technique was well known, and directions for the "cure" were sent to all medicine men who purchased stocks of a liniment called Modern Miracles. "Send one of your Company about town during the day looking for cripples for you to cure at night," suggested a

Modern Miracles flyer. "Have at least one each night. Either have a performer rub him in the dressing room while you are lecturing or rub him yourself on the open stage. If you rub as directed . . . you Will Make the CURE Then and There."[29]

Burt's liniment doctor, after one such spectacular stage cure in Illinois, neglected to leave town quickly enough, and was earnestly sought by an uncured and humiliated cripple with a gun. "The Doctor," said Burt, "forewarned and advised that the man was really dangerous, decided to get out of town, instructing the quartet to pack up and await him in La Salle." There was no train until late at night so the terrified pitchman set out cross-country on foot, carefully avoiding the main roads. "It was about midnight when the Doctor heard the barking of dogs coming in his direction. He pictured a posse, led by bloodhounds and he remembered the killer with the gun. Just ahead of him was a large apple tree and up he went to await the worst. And it came—a rabbit chased by a pair of rabbit-hounds passed directly under the tree. As they continued on their nocturnal rambling, he dropped to the ground and sought lodging at a small town a mile or so up the road." The experience had been too much for the already strained nerves of the liniment doctor, who went into a rapid emotional decline. "His lectures became feeble—at times, pitiful. He stumbled and stammered over the most simple words. His salesmanship became nil and business with the bottles dropped to practically nothing. He plowed back all the cash in his possession into a failing business and the show finally closed in Joplin, Missouri."[30]

A more fortunate Hamlin imitator was Doc C. M. Townsend, who traveled around Indiana and Ohio with a troupe that was widely known as the "Wizard Oil Company" even though it sold only Townsend's Magic Oil and other patent medicines bottled under the doctor's personal label.[31] Like the performers in legitimate Wizard Oil units, Townsend's company sang and played musical instruments from a wagon that doubled as a stage—the doctor himself played the B-flat cornet and his assistants joined in on the bass horn, bass drum, banjo, violin, and tuba. Townsend arranged his itinerary so that his vibrant blue and gold wagon would roll into each town just as school

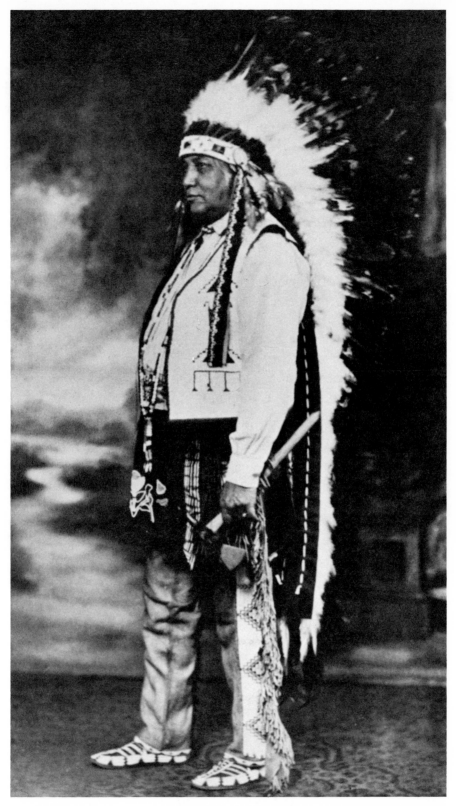

A medicine showman, Chief Sheet Lightning.

let out for the noon recess. Followed by a crowd of eager scholars, he would parade through the town with the band playing furiously to draw the curious away from their dinner tables. Bowing to right and left and doffing his top hat, Townsend would majestically scatter circulars into the crowd advertising his lectures and the elevating musical entertainments that accompanied them.[32]

In the fall of 1875, Townsend gained a new bass drummer in the person of James Whitcomb Riley, late of Doc McCrillis's Standard Remedies Company. "I shall never forget," Riley said, "how ashamed I was in Fortville to have a cousin of mine see me beating the bass drum with that show."[33] But shortly he was feeling more secure and content. The incident in Fortville was "but the blur of a moment," and in his letters home Riley began to create an idyll that ignored the discomforts and humiliations of medicine show life. To his friend John Skinner, Riley wrote grandly of the sleepy pace of life on the Magic Oil wagon and the feverish excitement of the show and sale:

> I am having first rate times considering the boys I am with. They, you know, are hardly my kind, but they are pleasant and agreeable and with Doctor Townsend for sensible talk occasionally, I have really a happy time. We sing along the road when we tire of talking, and when we tire of that and the scenery, we lay ourselves along the seats and dream the happy hours away as blissfully as the time honoured baby in the sugar trough. I shall not attempt an explicit description of all that I have passed through, but will give a brief outline. We "struck" Fortville first, as you already know—stayed over night and came near dying of loneliness. There is where I "squeeled" on street business, that is the portion of it where I was expected to bruise the bass drum. Well, I have been "in clover" ever since, and do what I please and when I please. I made myself thoroughly solid with "Doxy" (the playful patronymic I have given the doctor) by introducing a blackboard system of advertising which promises to be the best card out. I have two boards

about three feet by four, which during the street concert, I fasten on the sides of the wagon and letter and illustrate during the performance and through the lecture. There are dozens in the crowd that stay to watch the work going on that otherwise would drift away from the fold during the drier portion of the Doctor's harangue. Last night at Winchester I made a decided sensation by making a rebus of the well-known lines from Shakespeare—

"Why let pain your pleasure spoil,
For want of Townsend's Magic Oil?"—

with a life-sized bust of the author; and at another time a bottle of Townsend's Cholera Balm on legs, and a very bland smile on its cork, making a "Can't come in" gesture at the skeleton Death, who drops his scythe and hour glass to flee. Oh! I'm stared at like the fat woman on the side-show banner.[34]

Each new performance with Dr. Townsend was a romantic adventure to Riley. During fair week, billed as the "Hoosier Wizard," he felt his imagination liberated somehow as he scribbled away on his blackboard under the torches. "When the moon rose to blend her light with the decorations and costumes," Riley said, "I was transported to the land of the Arabian Nights. It was an Aladdin show."[35]

A similarly romantic view of medicine show life sent hundreds of young men on the road in the years that followed Riley's excursion with the Magic Oil troupe. In the last two decades of the nineteenth century, small-town boys like him— armed with a boundless confidence in the credulity of country people and a talent for creating an "Aladdin show"—eagerly transformed themselves into medicine showmen. The majority of them modeled their shows and their careers in the image of the two great Western medicine showmen, Healy and Bigelow, the proprietors of the famous Kickapoo Indian Sagwa.

5

THE
KICKAPOO IDEA

Kickapoo Indian Sagwa . . . is the only remedy
the Indians ever use, and has been known to
them for ages. An Indian would as soon be
without his horse, gun or blanket as without
Sagwa.

Colonel William F. Cody
in a Kickapoo testimonial

Buffalo Bill to the contrary, no American Indian had ever
heard of Kickapoo Indian Sagwa before 1881. In that year
Sagwa—followed by Kickapoo Indian Oil, Kickapoo Buffalo
Salve, Kickapoo Indian Cough Cure, and Kickapoo Indian
Worm Killer—sprang full-blown from the fertile imaginations
of a Connecticut Yankee and a would-be Western hero from
Bee County, Texas. The Kickapoo Indian Medicine Company,
founded by John Healy and Charles Bigelow, was certainly not
the first of the Indian medicine firms to send out shows, but
Healy and Bigelow's extraordinary promotional scheme was to
make them the largest and most prosperous turn-of-the-century medicine show advertisers and to inspire a host of admir-
ing imitators who toured the country with similar Indian performances.

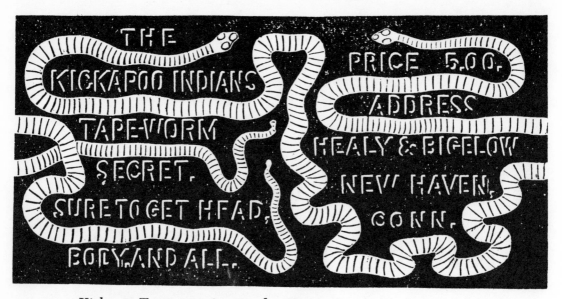

Kickapoo Tapeworm Secret advertisement.
BELLA C. LANDAUER COLLECTION, NEW-YORK HISTORICAL SOCIETY, NEW
YORK CITY.

John E. Healy, a small-time New Haven peddler, had been a
shoe salesman, a door-to-door vendor of vanishing cream, a
drummer boy in the Union army, and, after the war, entrepreneur of a liniment called King of Pain.[1] With the profits
from King of Pain, he launched himself as the proprietor of a
curious theatrical troupe, Healy's Hibernian Minstrels, a novelty variation of the popular blackface minstrel show. Ultimately Healy disbanded the minstrel company and joined
forces with Dr. E. H. Flagg, a Baltimore pitchman. Flagg, who
drew crowds with songs and violin solos, peddled a liniment
known as Flagg's Instant Relief from a suitcase on street corners. The formula for Flagg's Instant Relief, which was to become the basis for Kickapoo Indian Oil, included virtually the
same ingredients as the already famous Hamlin's Wizard Oil.[2]

In the fall of 1879 Healy and Flagg hired an assistant,
Charles Bigelow. Born on a farm in Bee County, Texas, just after the Mexican War, Bigelow rejected the plow for a chance to
tour with a bogus Indian medicine man, Phil Grant, known as
Dr. Yellowstone. Before long, Bigelow had created an exotic
frontier image for himself, complete with sombrero, shoulder-
length hair, the nickname of Texas Charlie, and a rapid-fire

stock of Indian medicine lore. In 1873 he was operating on a
less than modest scale in Baltimore, pitching herbs on street
corners. Business was poor and Bigelow and seven other pitchmen lived together for several months in two rooms that cost
them a total of four dollars a week.[3] Half a dozen years later
Bigelow's luck changed for good when he and Nevada Ned
Oliver were hired by Healy and Flagg to take out a four-man
troupe to advertise and sell liver pads and liniment. Nevada
Ned played the banjo and Texas Charlie, the "doctor," lectured on the merits of Healy and Flagg products and their vital importance to the health of the nation.

    Two years later they had three units on the road and Flagg
had disappeared from the company. It was then that Healy
came up with the idea that was to grow into the largest medicine show in America. Nevada Ned, who had left to travel
with a Percy Williams liver pad unit, was called to the Conti-
nental Hotel in Philadelphia. There Healy explained to him a
scheme for a new kind of medicine show: "His plan was to hire
a few Indians, rent a storeroom and have the medicine sim-
mering like a witch's brew in a great iron pot inside a tepee.
The brew of roots, herbs, and barks, refined from a formula
handed down through the generations, was to be ladled out to
the public, who would provide their own bottles."[4] Bigelow
objected to dispensing medicine by the dipperful, and a com-
promise was agreed upon: Healy, Bigelow, and eventually
Oliver, who was still under contract to Williams, were to become Indian agents who bottled and sold the remedies of the
Kickapoo tribe. The giant vat and the Indians would remain,
but only as atmosphere. Shortly, Healy and Bigelow opened in
a storeroom in a Providence hotel, with the Indians as background, but without a show. Their third stop that season was
Boston, where the first of the Kickapoo medicine shows was
produced in a tent pitched opposite the Boston and Providence
station. For the winter season the show moved into the old
Aquarium at Broadway and Thirty-fourth Street in New York,
and the Kickapoo Indian Medicine Company was fairly
launched.

    The partners shrouded all of the Kickapoo products in an
aura of mystery and romance. Not even Healy and Bigelow

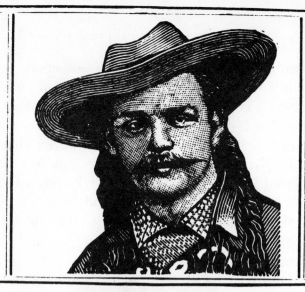

Pages from a free magazine given to customers of the Kickapoo Indian Medicine Company.

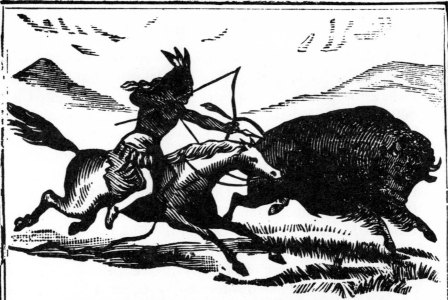

KICKAPOO INDIAN HUNTING BUFFALO FOR TALLOW TO MAKE KICKAPOO INDIAN SALVE.

KICKAPOO
INDIAN SALVE!

Made from Buffalo Tallow, combined with Healing Herbs and Barks.

It is a perfect cure-all in Skin Diseases—for the various forms of **Tetter**, dry, scaly, moist or itchy, for **Erysipelas**, recent or chronic; **Pimples or Bloches on the Face, Scald Head, Barber's Itch**, and all annoying, unsightly eruptions of the skin; also, painful soft **Corns**, and **Burns** and **Itching Piles**.

SOLD BY ALL DRUGGISTS.   **PRICE 25 CENTS.**

TRY IT!   *KEEP IT IN THE HOUSE!*

BONNETS ARE HIGH. A fashion journal says; "Bonnets come high this season." We do not remember when they did not, as any man who has been compelled to pay for them can testify.

themselves, said the advertisements, were privileged to know the formulas for Kickapoo products; the wary Indians, in fact, included a special element in each remedy which caused it to defy chemical analysis. The necessary roots, barks, gums, herbs, leaves, and buffalo fat were supposedly shipped East from the Kickapoo reservation to the Healy and Bigelow laboratories. There such exotic plants as Indian Star Root, Indian Dog Root, Indian Apple Plant, Indian Onion, Indian Bell, Squaw Flower, Prairie Weed, Indian Man Root, and Sa-wan-ka-wa Bark were combined in secret by the wisest of the Kickapoo Indian medicine men, who had left the reservation to serve Healy and Bigelow and the cause of health.[5] In fact, although the medicines sometimes included a few herbs gathered by Healy and Bigelow's Indians, they were chiefly made with materials purchased from quite ordinary and unromantic drug wholesalers.[6] In later years, Nevada Ned included the Sagwa recipe in a book of household hints he compiled. The recipe called for common combinations of roots, herbs, and alcohol, and produced a mild stomachic and laxative.[7] A rival healer ungenerously claimed, however, that Sagwa—"the only remedy the Indians ever use"—was originally compounded of aloes and stale beer.[8]

The company operated out of Boston from 1881 to 1884, when the headquarters was moved to New York. In 1887, Healy and Bigelow shifted the operation to New Haven, where Kickapoo was to remain for ten years until a final move to nearby Clintonville.[9] The Kickapoo building in New Haven, which the partners' circulars and magazines referred to as the "Principal Wigwam," or "Main Winter Quarters of the Kickapoo Indians," was part factory, part dormitory, part dime museum, and part craft shop.[10] Healy and Bigelow, both devoted followers of Barnum, decorated every spare inch of the building's exterior with an exotic collection of tepees, shields, spears, and other Indian paraphernalia, and invited the public to view their charges in a bizarre re-creation of their native habitat:

> Near by the river front on Grand Avenue, New Haven, Conn., stands a towering massive warehouse;

into this you are invited to visit the uncultured sons of the plain and forest, who assist in carrying on one of the most original enterprises on the continent. In the upper portions of the building these sons of the far west find a home; in fact, it is their hunting grounds (*pro tem.*), and if one will but shut one's eyes to the fact that a roof is between himself and heaven, there is little or nothing left for imagination. It is here the Indians are received prior to being consigned to their duties in the extensive factory or to encampments upon the road. Another portion of the building is occupied with tents erected and equipped exactly as though they formed a settlement on the plains. The clothing and food supplies of the band are scattered about with that unstudied elegance of disorder which, as the initiated are well aware, forms a great attraction to the free and easy red and pale faces, constituting the grandest charm of life away from the trammels of civilization.[11]

After passing through the rest of the warehouse, visitors were treated to a peep into the "private office (or *sanctum sanctorum*) of Messrs. Healy & Bigelow," a veritable museum of Indian curios, carpeted with the skins of wild animals and hung with a collection of relics, trophies, weapons and artifacts—each one certified as strictly genuine by the proprietors.[12]

By trading on the mystique of the Indian, Healy and Bigelow were following the lead of dozens of nineteenth-century quacks and patent medicine promoters.[13] It was the belief among many white Americans that the Indian was a natural physician, endowed with an iron constitution because he possessed secrets of healing unknown to the white man. This view was reinforced by the fact that a number of Indian botanicals had been adopted by white physicians and because the Indian had become a popular symbol of the strength and purity of the New World.[14] Quacks and patent medicine men, recognizing the possibilities of such a powerful emblem, borrowed the Indian and made him their own. So-called Indian doctors—many of them white practitioners of what was loosely termed

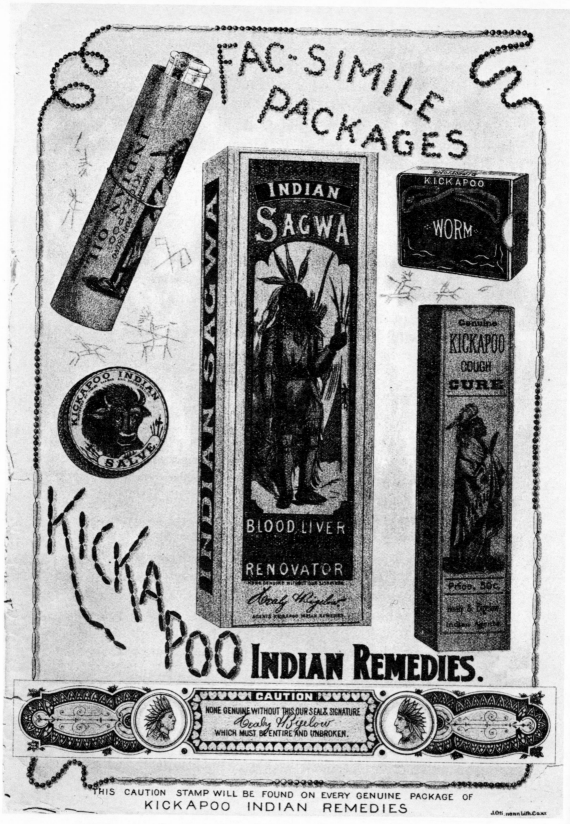

Kickapoo products. THEATRE COLLECTION, NEW YORK PUBLIC LIBRARY.

"Indian medicine" or "medicine according to Indian theory"—could be found in most large towns or riding country circuits.[15] Presses ground out a host of books which allegedly revealed to the reader the mysteries of Indian pharmacology: *The Indian Doctor's Dispensatory, The Indian Guide to Health, The North American Indian Doctor, or Nature's Method of Curing and Preventing Disease According to the Indians,* and many similar works capitalized on the power of the Indian medicine idea over those who shared the popular enthusiasm for botanic medicine or distrusted the educated white physician.[16] From patent medicine advertisements, labels, packages, and brochures, the Indian started out in awful solemnity, offering to the ailing the secrets of good health supposedly known only to the red man. For many it was clear that Indian remedies were not mere patent medicines, but, as the proprietor of one popular Indian tonic phrased it, "Nature's Gift to Nature's Children."[17]

By the late eighties a flood of almanacs, circulars, and magazines built around this bizarre vision of the Indian and his medicine was pouring from the Principal Wigwam in New Haven. The Wigwam was the symbolic home of the patron saint of Kickapoo advertising, Little Bright Eye, the Kickapoo Indian Princess:

> Prairie flower of grace and splendor,
> Little Bright Eye trips along!
> Oh! her glance so soft and tender,
> Thrills us as the birdie's song!
> O'er the wild and bounding prairie,
> Speeding like a young gazelle,
> Sunny hearted as a fairy,
> Beams the maiden loved so well.[18]

It was Little Bright Eye who presided over the pages of *The Indian Illustrated Magazine, Life and Scenes Among the Kickapoo Indians, The Kickapoo Indian Dream Book,* and other publications put out by the firm.[19] Patent medicine almanacs had been in use since the forties, but Healy and Bigelow expanded the idea into a whole line of free or inexpensive publications that mingled advertisements for their products with medical advice, testimonials, stories, jokes and useful information.[20]

Kickapoo publications were aimed at the Victorian family, and the partners were careful to preserve the appropriate tone. Temperance was promoted by the Chief of the Kickapoos, who announced to homemakers in thirty-two verses the virtues of clean living and Healy and Bigelow products:

> I am Chief of the Kickapoo Indian tribe
> And am strong as a brave can be,
> Not brandy, nor whiskey do I imbibe,
> Nor the Chinaman's poisonous tea.
>
> But Indian Sagwa I often do take,
> For it's good for man at least.
> It cures the body of many an ache,
> And stomach for many a feast.[21]

The preface to one edition of *Life and Scenes* announced that the magazine "will be found to differ somewhat from popular treatises on the subject of health, inasmuch as the diseases of the sexes are omitted. The reason of this omission is, that the book is intended to be placed on every table as a work of general interest and reference, and not to be under lock and key, as it contains nothing that the Head of any family need object to."[22] Ladies, however, could send for a special booklet on female complaints which was especially prepared for the fair sex by the redoubtable Little Bright Eye.[23]

A typical magazine, *Kickapoo Indians: Life and Scenes Among the Indians,* begins with a short piece called "Fleet-Footed Indians," followed by "The Red Hunters," a poem.[24] Next are biographical sketches of General Custer and Buffalo Bill, an article on the health of the Kickapoo Squaw, and a map showing the location of the Kickapoo Indian Reservation near Oklahoma City. Two articles, "The Indians' Knowledge of Nature's Remedies," and "The Medicine Chief," are followed by a short-short story, "The Broken Vow, or the Hunter's Dog." Next come "Burnt at the Stake," "Kit Carson's Double Victory," and "White Buffalo, the Sculptor's Friend." The writing in *Kickapoo Indians* is florid and overwrought ("Horrible to behold, dreadful to relate!"), and is reminiscent of the prose of Nevada Ned Oliver, who was the author of such popular adventure novels as *Mexican Bill, the Cowboy Detective,* and *The King of Gold; the Mystery of the Lost Mine.*[25] It may well be that many of the pieces, which were used over and over for years, were originally written by Oliver during his association with Healy and Bigelow.

In their magazines, Healy and Bigelow were turning themselves into frontier heroes. The old raw West was rapidly dying out, replaced by a picturesque literary and theatrical West created by popular authors, showmen, and publicists. Healy and Bigelow, like Buffalo Bill Cody, were products of the nostalgia that accompanied the closing of the frontier; and like Cody their reputation as heroic Western figures was chiefly the result of a carefully conceived public relations campaign. It was Bigelow on whom the official Kickapoo publications lavished the most attention, celebrating his exploits in a flood of pictures, stories, and doggerel verse. In "Texas Charlie," for example, Bigelow was portrayed skimming over the prairie somewhat in the manner of Little Bright Eye:

> Hurrah! once more the prairies wide
> Are bounding 'neath my feet.
> My gallant steed again I stride,
> His step is lightning fleet.
> The breath of morn is in the sky
> And free as eagle's wing,
> While on the trail I gaily fly,
> My merry song to sing.[26]

Perhaps the most favored official anecdote about Texas Charlie concerned his supposed discovery of Sagwa. The story was reprinted countless times with minor variations in detail, under such titles as "Snatched From the Jaws of Death: Texas Charlie's Thrilling Story of His Delivery From Sickness By the Indians," or "Sagwa's Surprising Story: How Texas Charlie's Life Was Saved By the Indians." The latter piece (subtitled "The Adventures of a United States Government Scout. The same Remedy that effected his cure now used throughout the Civilized World") is a typical Healy and Bigelow humbug:

Some years ago, Mr. Chas. Bigelow, now one of the proprietors of the famous Kickapoo Indian Remedies, was acting as a government scout in the Indian territory. He was known at that time as "Texas Charlie," and while on one of his expeditions was taken sick with a severe fever, and for a few days lay at death's door. During his sickness he was cared for by an Indian Chief and his family, in whose lodge he lay, so weak he could hardly raise his eyelids. An Indian doctor visited him, and gave him that now most famous of Indian remedies, Indian Sagwa, and by its use he was snatched from the jaws of death and restored to health, owing his life to the wonderful efficacy and curative power of this medicine. He then endeavored to persuade the Indians to give him the secret of its ingredients. This at first they refused to do, but after much persuasion and many discussions they at last partially yielded to his request, and the Chief of the Tribe sent East with Mr. Bigelow five of his most renowned medicine men, together with an ample supply of the roots, herbs, barks, gums, etc., used in the manufacture of their medicines. What started thus in a small way has ever since increased, and today there is manufactured from similar materials gathered by the Indians themselves, their famous remedies, which have done so much to alleviate suffering of every description.[27]

The shows created by Healy and Bigelow represented another phase of the same frontier mumbo jumbo that dominated the stories and poems in the Kickapoo magazines. The result was a portrait of the Indian that bore as little relationship to reality as the creations of James Fenimore Cooper and the nineteenth-century stage Indian, both of which were described by Mark Twain as belonging to "an extinct tribe that never existed."[28] Healy and Bigelow were to resurrect that tribe once again, tailor-making the Kickapoo Indian to their own unique specifications and setting him about the task of peddling patent medicine.

6

THE KICKAPOO SHOWS

In Order to Portray to the Civilized World
Genuine Scenes in Indian Life, Messrs. Healy
& Bigelow, the Eastern Agents of the Kickapoo
Indians, have, at an enormous outlay, perfected
arrangements whereby they will be enabled to
make A GRAND TOUR OF THE UNITED
STATES, VISITING THE PRINCIPAL CITIES
AND TOWNS, Bringing with them their Squaws,
Medicine Men AND PAPPOOSES [sic], En-
camping out in the Summer Time in their Wig-
wams and Tents, As they do on the Plains, And
in the Winter time in Public Halls.

Life and Scenes Among the Kickapoo Indians

The immediate origin of the Kickapoo shows lay in the Indian
performances which had been produced for years by white
showmen. Americans had always been curious about Indian
life and customs, and exhibitions of dances and ceremonies
had been popular since the seventeenth century. At first, Indian performers were treated with reasonable courtesy. When
a group of Cherokee warriors and chiefs, on a visit to New York
in 1768, agreed to perform a war dance on stage at the John
Street Theatre, a cautious manager warned the public about

the respect due the performers: "It is humbly presumed, that no Part of the Audience will forget the proper Decorum so essential to all public Assemblies, particularly on this Occasion, as the Persons who have condescended to contribute to their Entertainment are of Rank and Consequence in their own Country."[1] By the nineteenth century, however, Indians had been reduced by showmen to dime museum novelties, and the performances developed by museum operators often concentrated on the most sanguinary aspects of Indian life. A show presented at Peale's Museum in 1827, for example, was designed to produce a pleasant tingle of fear in white spectators when a group of Iroquois demonstrated "the manner in which they skulk and lay [sic] in ambush and the manner of scalping an enemy," and the "ceremonies used on the return of the victorious warriors; presenting spoils taken in war to the head Chiefs of the Tribe; grand war dance, the war-whoop will be given as they rush on the enemy."[2]

By the early eighties the Indian show had been transformed by Colonel William F. Cody into Buffalo Bill's Wild West and by Healy and Bigelow into the Kickapoo Indian medicine shows. The Wild West show as it was developed by Cody and Pawnee Bill was generally a far more elaborate production than the Kickapoo entertainments. But both were aimed at the popular taste for romantic and sensational versions of the "Indian troubles" making headlines in the eighties and early nineties. As in the dime novel and the melodrama, the result was an ambiguous vision of the Indian, who combined a dignity and natural wisdom denied the white man with a disposition naturally inclined to all that was dark, cold, and treacherous. Healy and Bigelow's Indians were clearly the villains of the piece, shown attacking wagon trains and massacring settlers in a frenzied blood lust. But in the same shows the Kickapoos were also displayed compounding healing remedies to be dispensed to their hated enemy the white man. In the Healy and Bigelow version, the Indian became whatever he needed to be at the moment—perpetrator of lurid and bloodcurdling acts of cruelty or benign and lofty forest creature from the patent medicine labels.

Before 1890, Healy and Bigelow claimed to have almost eight hundred Indians in their employ, either compounding medi-

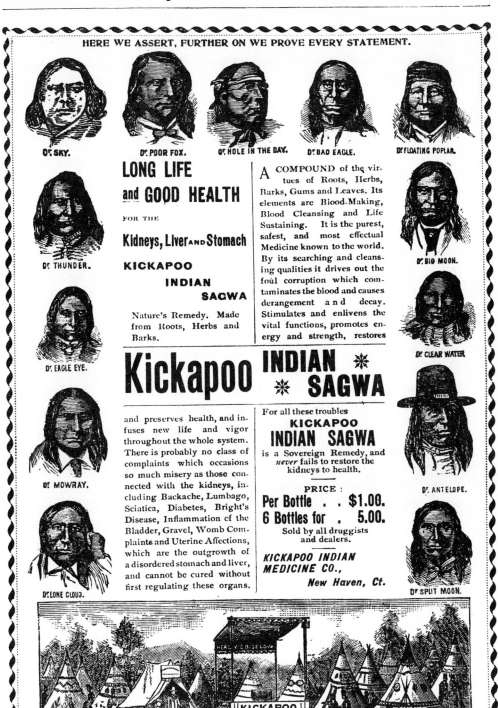

Indians who performed with Kickapoo Indian Medicine Company shows and a Kickapoo encampment.

THEATRE COLLECTION, NEW YORK PUBLIC LIBRARY.

cine in New Haven or traveling with the various units of the Kickapoo show.[3] Fifty "medical men" acted as the Indians' agents. Many of the agents, the partners said, were well-known scouts and former Indian fighters "who by their bravery in war have obtained such ascendancy over the Red Man that they willingly yield to their control."[4] The veiled hint of potential uprising, only forestalled by the courage of the Kickapoo Indian agents, was undoubtedly conceived to add spice to the actual appearance of the braves around the mysterious bubbling pot of Sagwa at shows or marching, single file, down Main Street to pose in front of some small-town drugstore.

The stalwarts of the Kickapoo performances, whose somber faces appeared in a thousand advertisements and magazine illustrations, included Dove Wing, Thunder Cloud, Ma-Chu-Ta-Ga, Poor Fox, Antelope, Mowray, Clear Water, and Floating Poplar. If they had a common bond, it lay in the fact that none of them were really Kickapoos. The first Indians hired by the firm were Chief Thunder Cloud and seven other braves of the Caughnawagas, a subdivision of the Iroquois from the south bank of the Saint Lawrence above Montreal.[5] Over the years, most of Healy and Bigelow's so-called Kickapoos were from small bands of New York Iroquois and Canadian Indians, together with a mixture of Pawnees, Crees, Sioux, Blackfeet, Chippewas, Cherokees, and Peruvian Indians.[6] In some cases Healy and Bigelow contracted with federal Indian agents for their performers, offering thirty dollars a month and room and board to their wards.[7] As many as two hundred Indians at a time were delivered straight from their reservations to the Principal Wigwam. To swell the ranks, however, the partners were not averse to hiring away Indians from Buffalo Bill's Wild West or employing Indian impersonators, including two Dubliners named Leary and Connor.[8] Meanwhile, the real Kickapoo Indians, desperate and bitter enemies of the white man, sulked on the barren Deep Fork Reservation in Indian Territory, which Healy and Bigelow's advertising described as a veritable Garden of Eden inhabited by a race of benevolent primitive physicians.[9]

The traveling Kickapoo Indian villages, as Healy and Bigelow described them, were almost as idyllic as the Oklahoma reservation. A visit to a Kickapoo encampment, the partners said, was equal to a lesson in natural history: "Their camp grounds are as picturesque as they would be on the plains. They have some interesting relics to show you, and can entertain you in good shape. You can watch them compounding their medicines, carefully sorting the various barks, roots, and herbs which form the chief ingredients of the famous Sagwa. They have many interesting books written by themselves, giving you a pictorial account of their life on the plains, which they will have pleasure in making you a present of."[10] For the children there was a model encampment, the "Wonderful Wild West and Kickapoo Indian Paper Doll Camp," which neatly grafted Buffalo Bill, astride a paper charger, onto the typical Kickapoo Indian village.[11]

Over the years, Kickapoo Indian villages came in all sizes and degrees of extravagance. The smallest traveling units, like Kickapoo Camp Number Fifteen, consisted only of an agent, several Indians, and a few performers. "Our harmonious working company," wrote the Indian agent, R. S. Palmer, "may their shadows never grow lean. Our team (horses) are the pets of the company—Dick and Charley. Our Indians are: —Ogalia Fire. Princess Red Fire and Brave Bear. Our artists, E. Thorn, H. Cushing, and Thomas Clannon."[12] At the other end of the scale was the stationary show created for Healy and Bigelow in Chicago by Nevada Ned, which included in its company twenty-five Indians, one hundred and ten performers, picked up cheaply from a stranded carnival, and two brass bands.[13]

The standard Kickapoo camp, however, was designed to be run by a company of ten to twenty and consisted of half a dozen tepees, several tents used by the Indian agent, a twenty-foot-wide portable covered stage, and a few Gale's Patent Beacon Lights. Units also carried the equipment necessary to present balloon ascensions during the day and fireworks displays at night.[14] In the winter Kickapoo troupes would move into local halls and opera houses, confining their outdoor performances to street parades. A photograph of one of the summer villages, playing at Manchester Depot, Vermont, in 1885, shows the stage at one end of a rather crudely constructed roofless tent, with its side walls rolled up. Nearby are the ever

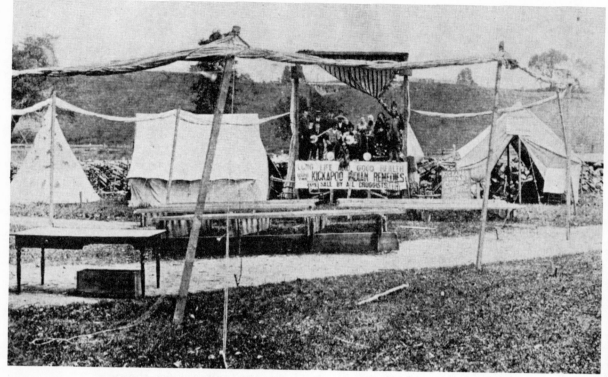

Kickapoo Indian Medicine Company encampment at Manchester Depot, Vermont, 1885.

present tepees, and tents used as consulting rooms by the Indian agent-doctor, who also managed the unit and lectured during the performance.

The Kickapoo Indian agent was a first-rate talker and a natural salesman. Carl Sandburg attended the Kickapoo shows once or twice each week during the six weeks or so that a unit played in Galesburg, Illinois, each year. Sandburg was transfixed by the sight of the Indians "stomping and howling their lonesome war songs," and by the eloquence of the lecturers, whose spiels for Sagwa and Kickapoo Indian Oil were imitated by the boys of the town for weeks afterwards.[15] The approaches varied. An aggressive agent, of patriarchal appearance, badgered and harangued his audience, calling down the "torments of seventeen devils on the head of anyone who dared to go away without a bottle."[16] Others affected a low-key bedside manner with crowds: "The pause, then the whispered diagnosis—*Kidney Trouble*, or *Cruel Dyspepsia*, or *Consumption the Killer*."[17]

In 1883 Nevada Ned Oliver acted as Indian agent for just the sort of unit that played Manchester Depot. Nevada Ned's unit carried six Indians and the same number of vaudeville performers, all of whom probably posted bills, called on druggists, and pitched and tore down the tent as medicine show people were expected to do. "The show," wrote Nevada Ned, "customarily began with the introduction of each of the Indians by name, together with some personal history. The stage setting was simple—an open platform with an Indian panorama in oils as a backdrop."[18] In front of the panorama sat the Indians in a half circle. "Five of the six would grunt acknowledgements; the sixth would make an impassioned speech in Kickapoo, interpreted by me; all made authentic by my scout habiliments and air of dignity . . . It was a most edifying oration as I translated it. What the brave actually said, I never knew, but I had reason to fear that it was not the noble discourse of my translation, for even the poker faces of his fellow savages sometimes were convulsed."[19] Nevada Ned lectured next, extolling the merits of Sagwa from the end of a runway that extended from the stage into the center of the audience. As the lecture ended the Indians beat fiercely on their tom-toms, the musicians played and Oliver dispensed Sagwa to the crowd. After the sale came a vaudeville show, interrupted for as many additional sales pitches as traffic would bear.

The first Kickapoo performances were often conventional Indian shows. One early unit under the direction of Texas Charlie Bigelow presented a show which consisted of "INDIAN MEDICINE MEN, INDIAN WAR DANCING, Indian Marriage Ceremonies, Indians Making Medicine, INDIAN SCENERY, INDIAN SONGS, Indian Curiosities," and an "INDIAN LECTURE."[20] The major attraction was a moving panorama—perhaps the same one used by Nevada Ned—which offered a whole Baedeker of the Wild West. Included on the five thousand feet of "Moving Canvas" painted by Orren C. Richards, a Boston scenic artist,

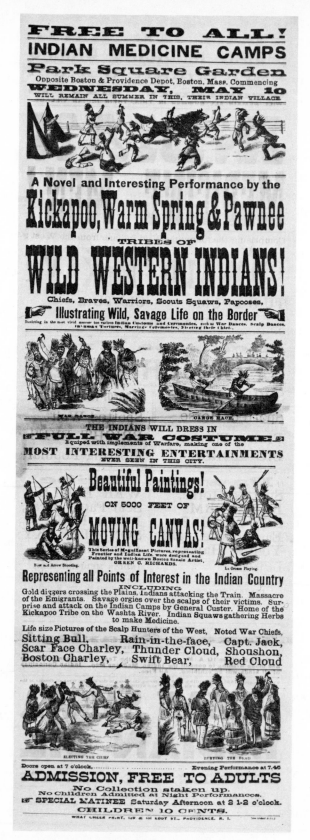

Early Kickapoo encampment poster.

Early Kickapoo encampment poster, verso.

THEATRE COLLECTION, HARVARD UNIVERSITY.

were "all points of Interest in the Indian Country," including such scenes as: "Gold diggers crossing the Plains, Indians attacking the Train. Massacre of the Emigrants. Savage orgies over the scalps of their victims. Surprise and attack on the Indian Camps by General Custer. Home of the Kickapoo Tribe on the Washta River. Indian Squaws gathering Herbs to make Medicine."[21]

Other units gradually began to include vaudeville turns along with the mock powwows and war dances. A unit that included half a dozen Indians and five white entertainers played for six nights at the town hall in Colebrook, New Hampshire, during the winter of 1907–8. Their show, which was interrupted about four times during an hour and a half for medicine pitches, consisted of singing, dancing, acrobatics, a chalk talk, a fire-eater, and several afterpieces. As a special added attraction, patrons were treated to an early motion picture, *The Dream of the Rarebit Fiend*.[22] A larger unit, with a dozen performers and probably as many Indians, played for nine weeks in Albany, New York, during the summer of 1883. Their programs and reviews were pasted into a scrapbook by a young boy named Townsend Walsh.[23] From early in May until the middle of July, when they moved on to Troy, the Kickapoo Indian Village was to be found on the Albany circus grounds, resolutely holding its own against such competition as George H. Adams's New Humpty Dumpty Ballet and Specialty Company, Doris's Inter-Ocean Circus, and Adam Forepaugh's famous circus. During the day the Indian agents provided free consultations and a line of Kickapoo products at their office tent. At two-thirty on Wednesdays and Saturdays and eight o'clock every night came the main show—admission ten cents, reserved seats an additional dime—in a three-thousand-seat tent grandly billed as "the only boarded floor pavilion in this or any other country—everything comfortable—four electric lights."

Townsend Walsh apparently attended the Indian village seven times during its nine-week stay in Albany, and the programs that he saved form a good account of the sort of entertainment provided by a large Kickapoo unit. The shows were ordinarily made up of ten or a dozen acts, probably inter-

PICTURESQUE
INDIAN VILLAGE!

ON CIRCUS LOT,
Cor. HUDSON AVE. and SWAN ST.,

Every Night at 8 O'Clock, and Wednesday and Saturday Afternoons at 2:30 O'Clock.

PROGRAMME.

1. A Sight of a Life-Time.

A group of Indian Men and Women in their native Songs and Dances, with an interesting Lecture on their ways, customs and habits, by

TEXAS CHARLIE.

2. Classic Groupings.

LEVANION, LEXINGTON AND JOHNSON.

3. MARINE CABLE WIRE,

MR. GEORGE LA ROSE.

4. INDIAN MEDICINE CEREMONY

Introducing the Horse and Buffalo Dance.

5. Fancy Rifle Shooting,

Holding the Rifle in twenty different positions, by the noted Scout and Indian Fighter, TEXAS CHARLIE. The Rifle used is from the celebrated Wesson Rifle Co,, of Worcester, Mass.

6. Contortion Act,

By the celebrated Indian Artist, GUS JOHNSON.

7. EMPRESS OF THE AIR,

MISS MAUD OSWALD, on the Flying Rings. Ladies and Children need have no fear for Miss Oswald's safety, as she is quite at home in the air.

8. Indian Marriage Ceremony.

9. Exercises on the Horizontal Bar,

LA ROSE BROS., LEVANION AND LEXINGTON.
CLOWN LEVANION.

The World's Greatest Canine Instructor, the original and only

10 Prof. HARRY M. PARKER,

And his Wonderful New Mastodon Dog Circus. The best trained Dogs on earth. 10 Large Handsome Dogs 10. Introducing large English Greyhounds, Setters, Spaniels, Tans, French, Russian, and Italian Poodles. 2 GREAT CLOWN DOGS. The Funniest Animals on Earth, who will keep the audience in a roar of laughter from beginning to the finish of the act. 8 Wonderful Leaping Dogs 8. Including the Great Royal English Greyhounds FLY, HANLON, and NELGIER who leap a distance of 30 feet and a height of 15 feet. A truly wonderful performance.

Introducing his wonderful leaping cat SPOT, springing 15 feet high through a hoop of fire.

The entertainment will conclude with ALFRED LEVANION'S Laughable Pantomime,

The Indian Village Beauty.

Char— —ic —mpany.

Showbill, Kickapoo encampment, Albany, New York, 1883.

rupted three or four times for medicine pitches. Each show be-
gan with the same Indian act: "A Sight of a Life Time! A
Group of Indian Men and Women in their Native Songs and
Dances." Near the beginning of the run the Indians were followed by Mr. and Mrs. Charles Fox in fancy rifle shooting;
Victor Laicelle, doing tumbling and balancing; the Howard
Sisters, with songs and dances; and a ventriloquist, Henderson,
the Man of Many Voices. After Henderson's act the Indians returned for a medicine ceremony, followed by Lexington,
Levanian, and Johnson, "in their New Sensational Aerial Act,
entitled Zampillerostation!"; Gilson and Miles, who were billed
as refined Irish comedians; and Miss Maude Oswald, the
"Greatest Female Aerial Artist in the World." After an Indian
courting scene the entire company returned for an afterpiece,
"Rooms to Rent."

In order to play for a number of weeks in a single town, a
Kickapoo unit was continually forced to vary its fare, announcing the weekly change of program in showbills and newspaper advertisements. The second time that Walsh attended a
performance, the bills show that Mr. and Mrs. Fox, Henderson,
Victor Laicelle, the Howard Sisters, and Gilson and Miles were
gone. Some were not to reappear again, but others, who probably moved to another Kickapoo unit for a few weeks, were
year-round employees of the firm who would return to Albany
as needed later in the run. Texas Charlie, blithely billed as the
champion rifle shot of the world, was narrating "A Sight of a
Life Time!" and giving displays of marksmanship. The La Rose
Brothers, acrobats, had joined the company, and Gus Johnson
of Lexington, Levanian, and Johnson, now billed as the "celebrated Indian Artist," was giving a solo contortion act. Professor Harry M. Parker and his New Mastadon [sic] Dog Circus
were also part of the company, with the "World's Greatest
Canine Instructor" displaying English greyhounds, setters,
spaniels, tans, and French, Russian, and Italian poodles, as
well as a cat named Spot that sprang fifteen feet in the air
through a hoop of fire. The Indian scenes remained the same,
but the afterpiece was changed to a comic pantomime called
"The Indian Village Beauty."

Throughout the remainder of their Albany run, the Kickapoo

unit presented virtually every sort of attraction. During the week in which the company showed against Doris's Inter-Ocean Circus, the Orren Richards panorama or a version of it made its appearance. Later there were aerial acts, a great deal of Irish and blackface comedy, and such exotic novelties as a midget Dutch comic, the "Skatorial Songsters," who performed while gliding around the stage on roller skates, and Jackley, "the only table performer on earth," who turned somersaults on a pile of tables that extended twenty-five feet in the air.

If the combination of burning wagon trains and blackface minstrel routines was somewhat eccentric, no one seems to have cared or even noticed—especially not Healy and Bigelow, who refused to trouble themselves about complex artistic questions so long as the Kickapoo shows continued to attract crowds and sell medicine. The Healy and Bigelow format worked well. For a dozen years or more after the founding of the company, the number of shows sent out by Kickapoo increased. By 1888 there were thirty-one units in the Chicago territory alone, and the total number of troupes on the road in the United States, Canada, and occasionally the West Indies, may have reached one hundred in some years before the turn of the century.[24] By the mid-eighties dozens of competing Indian medicine shows had appeared. Most were relatively small single-unit affairs made up of a few Indians (frequently Sioux obtained from reservations with the consent of the government), several performers, and the owner-lecturer, who generally claimed some sort of romantic Western background.[25] Among the proprietors were white "Indian doctors," self-styled frontier heroes, ex-Indian fighters, and some genuine Indians. Not a few were former employees of the Kickapoo Indian Medicine Company, and their shows were strongly influenced by Healy and Bigelow's Barnumesque ideas about organization and promotion.

7

INDIAN SHOWS AND SHOWMEN

"I struck Fisher Hill, Arkansas," said he, "in a buckskin suit, moccasins, long hair and a thirty-carat diamond ring that I got from an actor in Texarkana. I don't know what he ever did with the pocket knife I swapped him for it.

"I was Dr. Waugh-hoo, the celebrated Indian medicine man. I carried only one best bet just then, and that was Resurrection Bitters. It was made of life-giving plants and herbs accidentally discovered by Ta-qua-la, the beautiful wife of the chief of the Choctaw Nation, while gathering truck to garnish a platter of boiled dog for the annual corn dance."

O. Henry, "Jeff Peters as a Personal Magnet"

A number of Indian showmen gleefully adopted the Kickapoo name for their own shows and products. Some independent shows that claimed to be Kickapoo units peddled "Sagwah" or "Awaga" or another product with a name similar to that of Healy and Bigelow's best-selling tonic; others counterfeited Kickapoo labels or refilled old Sagwa bottles with their own preparations. Many imitated the kind of show presented by Kickapoo units, often on a low level. The genuine Kickapoo shows gave crowds good entertainment and remedies which, if nothing else, were at least innocuous. Their relatively good reputation meant that it was possible to play the same areas year after year, often remaining in small towns for at least a week and in large cities for months at a time. Fly-by-night imitators, however, usually provided poor entertainment and worse medicine, and often depended on a hasty exit from an outraged territory, "burning the lot" before moving on to a new area. The result was that Healy and Bigelow lost both money and goodwill because of cheap companies that represented themselves as Kickapoo units, and under the ominous headline, "Caution to the Public," the partners solemnly warned readers of their advertising matter against low-quality imitations manufactured by "Parties without Principle or Honor."[1]

The simplest form of Indian show was presented by the medicine pitchman who, though he may never have been closer to an Indian than those on exhibit at Buffalo Bill's Wild West, donned fringed buckskins and a war bonnet to pitch his cough cure or natural vegetable salve. One Dr. Newall—probably a white man—who called himself "the Native Indian Doctor," traveled about distributing handbills in which he respectfully offered his services "in the Original Indian Healing Art, to the sick and afflicted in this vicinity."[2] Dr. Newall could be found at his "Indian Encampment"—the exact place left blank on the handbill, to be filled in at each town on the doctor's tour—where he dispensed cures for "Costiveness, Indigestion, Dyspepsia, Flatulency, Headache, Cold Stomach, Cough, Pain in the Stomach, Jaundice, Dropsy, Stranguary, &c." The knowledge of the Indian physician, the doctor seemed to suggest in his advertising, had divine origins: "The Great Spirit is kind— he has taught his creatures what is good for them.—The real Natives of America have learned many good Medicines from the Beasts, Fowls, Fishes, and even from the insignificant insects themselves." In spite of such divine inspiration, Newall

THE TRADE CARD

Something For Nothing

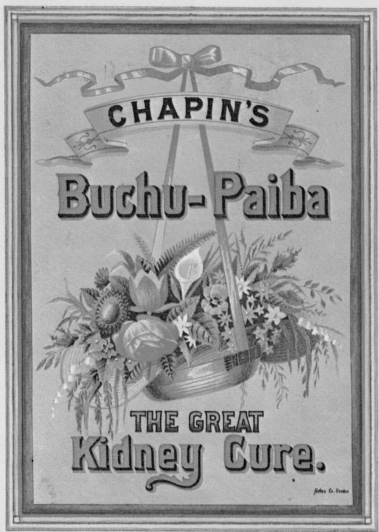

DURING THE EIGHTIES AND NINETIES, MEDICINE SHOWS AND DRUG STORES PRESENTED CUSTOMERS WITH AN ESPECIALLY POPULAR FREE SOUVENIR, THE TRADE OR ADVERTISING CARD. THE CARDS WERE WIDELY COLLECTED AND WERE OFTEN PASTED INTO ALBUMS, MANY OF WHICH SURVIVE TODAY IN MUSEUMS AND PRIVATE COLLECTIONS. ❧❧ THE ADVERTISING CARDS REPRODUCED HERE ARE FROM THE WILLIAM HELFAND COLLECTION.

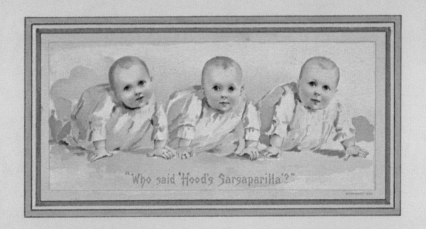

"Who said 'Hood's Sarsaparilla'?"

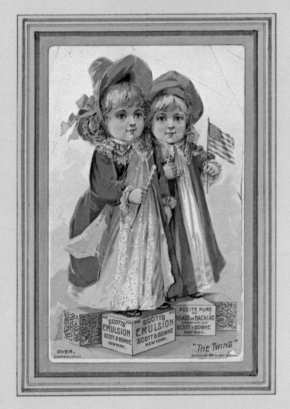

"The Twins"

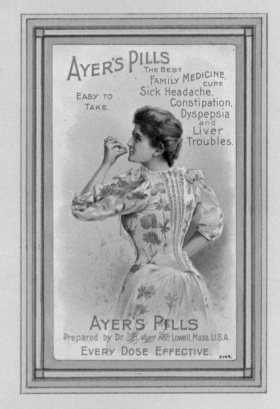

AYER'S PILLS
EASY TO TAKE.
THE BEST FAMILY MEDICINE, CURE Sick Headache, Constipation, Dyspepsia and Liver Troubles.

AYER'S PILLS
Prepared by Dr. J. C. Ayer & Co., Lowell, Mass. U.S.A.
EVERY DOSE EFFECTIVE.

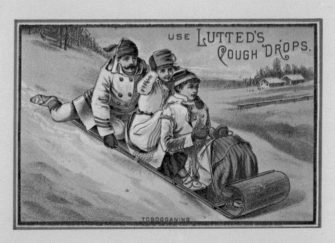

USE LUTTED'S COUGH DROPS.

TOBOGGANING

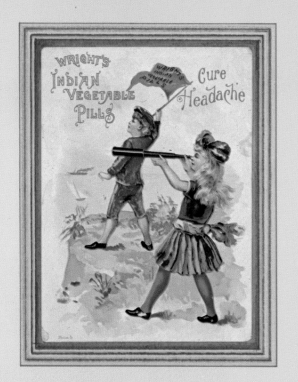

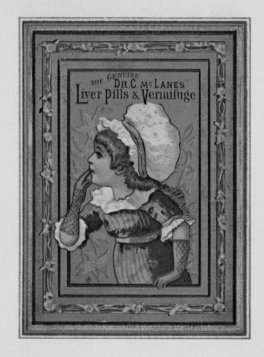

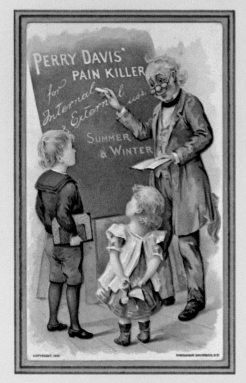

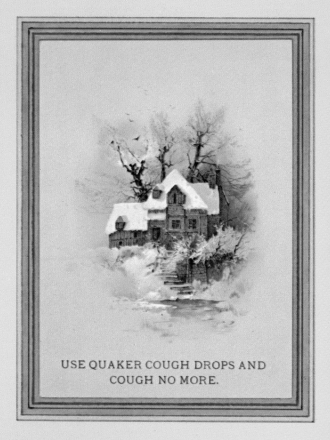

USE QUAKER COUGH DROPS AND
COUGH NO MORE.

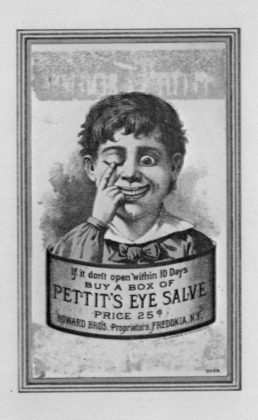

If it don't open within 10 Days
BUY A BOX OF
PETTIT'S EYE SALVE
PRICE 25¢
HOWARD BROS. Proprietors, FREDONIA, N.Y.

OVER.

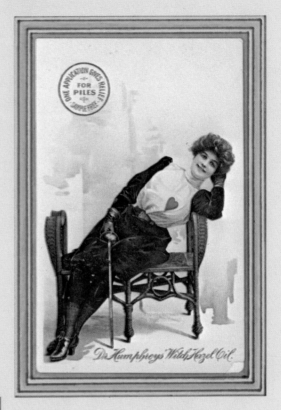

FOR PILES
ONE APPLICATION GIVES RELIEF
SAMPLE FREE

Dr Humphreys' Witch Hazel Oil.

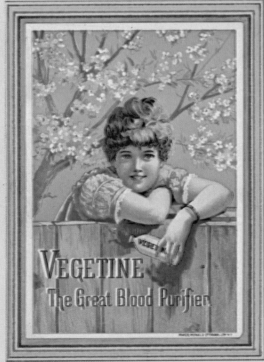

VEGETINE
The Great Blood Purifier.

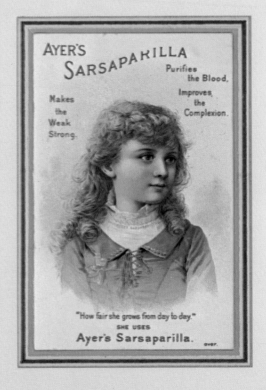

AYER'S
SARSAPARILLA

Makes
the
Weak
Strong.

Purifies
the Blood.
Improves
the
Complexion.

"How fair she grows from day to day."
SHE USES
Ayer's Sarsaparilla.

over.

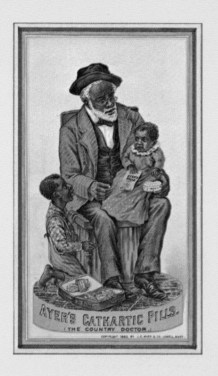

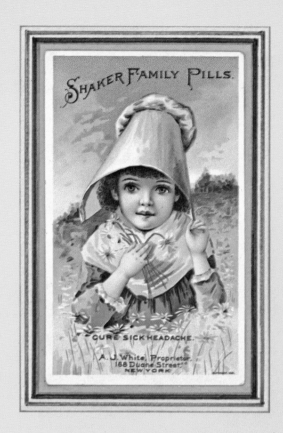

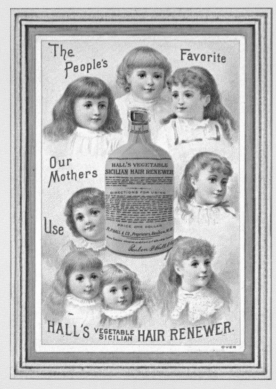

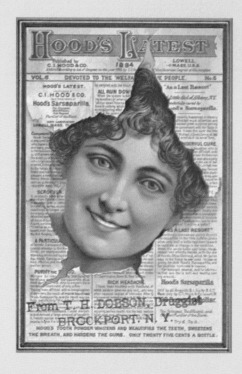

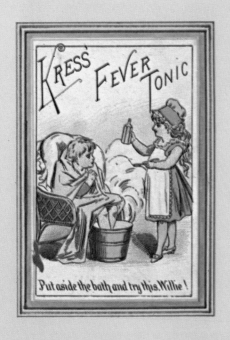

Kress' Fever Tonic

Put aside the bath and try this, Willie!

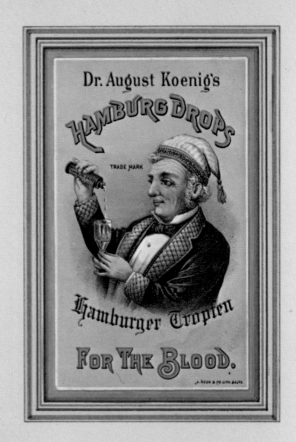

Dr. August Koenig's Hamburg Drops

TRADE MARK

Hamburger Tropfen

For The Blood.

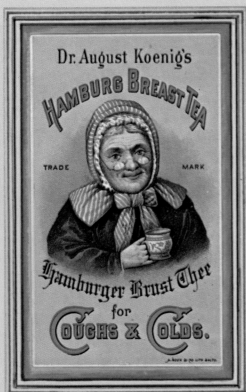

Dr. August Koenig's Hamburg Breast Tea

TRADE MARK

Hamburger Brust Thee for Coughs & Colds.

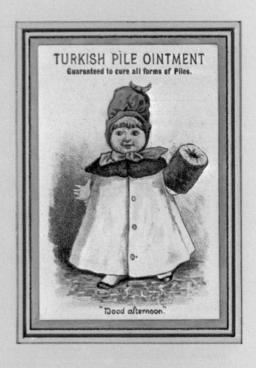

TURKISH PILE OINTMENT
Guaranteed to cure all forms of Piles.

"Good afternoon."

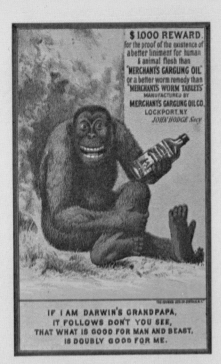
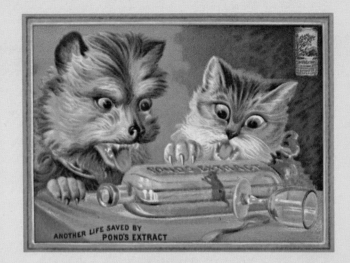

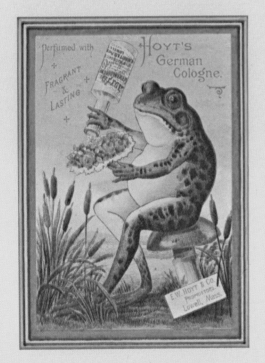
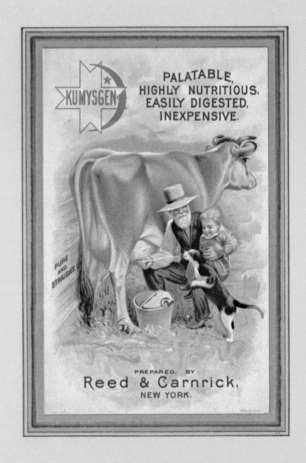

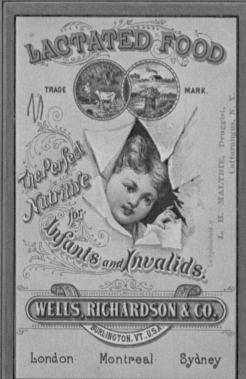

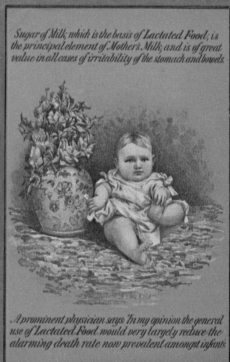

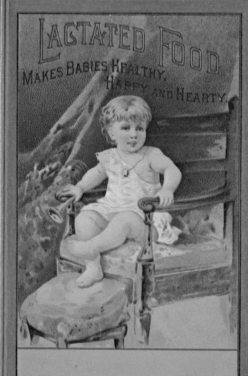

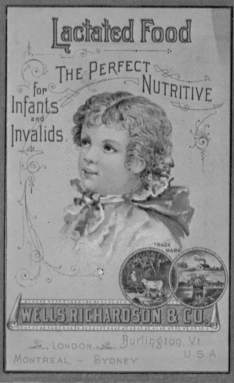

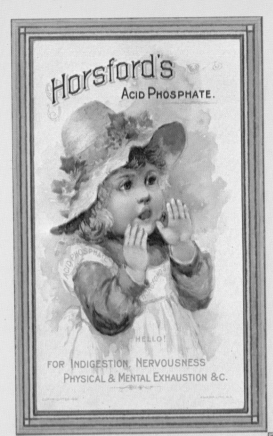

Horsford's
ACID PHOSPHATE.

HELLO!

FOR INDIGESTION, NERVOUSNESS
PHYSICAL & MENTAL EXHAUSTION &C.

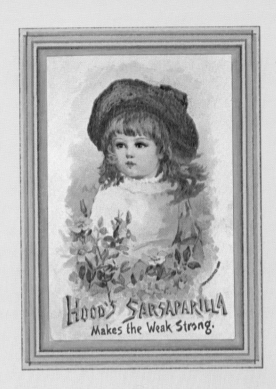

HOOD'S SARSAPARILLA
Makes the Weak Strong.

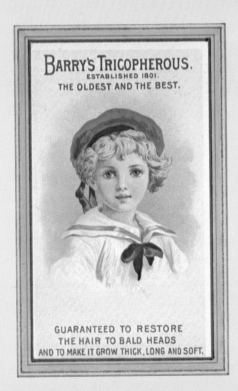

BARRY'S TRICOPHEROUS.
ESTABLISHED 1801.
THE OLDEST AND THE BEST.

GUARANTEED TO RESTORE
THE HAIR TO BALD HEADS
AND TO MAKE IT GROW THICK, LONG AND SOFT.

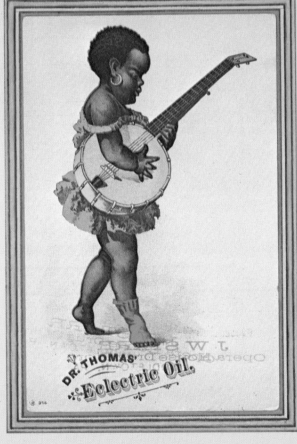

DR. THOMAS'
Eclectric Oil.

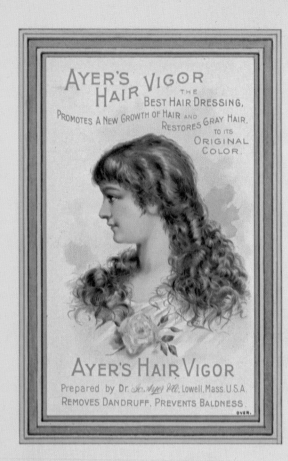

AYER'S HAIR VIGOR
THE BEST HAIR DRESSING,
PROMOTES A NEW GROWTH OF HAIR AND RESTORES GRAY HAIR,
TO ITS ORIGINAL COLOR.

AYER'S HAIR VIGOR

Prepared by Dr. J. C. Ayer & Co., Lowell, Mass. U.S.A.
REMOVES DANDRUFF, PREVENTS BALDNESS.
OVER.

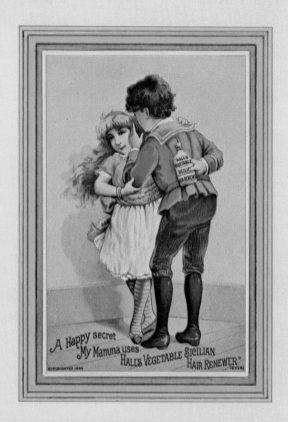

A Happy secret
"My Mamma uses HALL'S VEGETABLE SICILIAN HAIR RENEWER."
(OVER.)

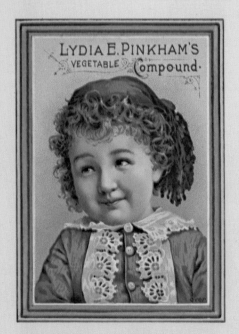

LYDIA E. PINKHAM'S
VEGETABLE Compound.

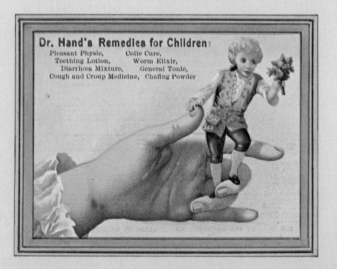

Dr. Hand's Remedies for Children:
Pleasant Physic,   Colic Cure,
Teething Lotion,   Worm Elixir,
Diarrhœa Mixture,   General Tonic,
Cough and Croup Medicine, Chafing Powder

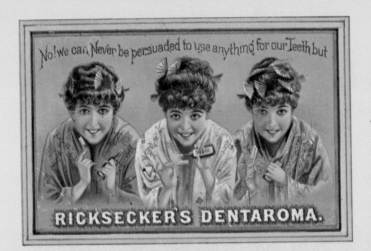

No! we can Never be persuaded to use anything for our Teeth but

RICKSECKER'S DENTAROMA.

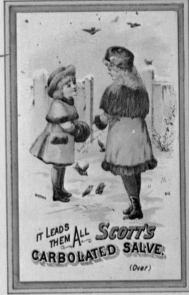

IT LEADS THEM ALL **SCOTT'S**
CARBOLATED SALVE.

(Over)

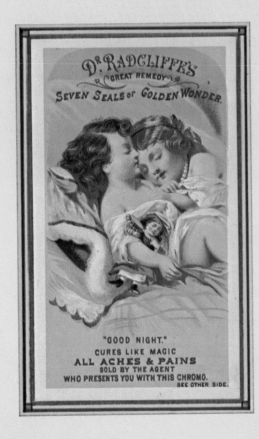

D.R. RADCLIFFE'S
GREAT REMEDY

SEVEN SEALS or GOLDEN WONDER.

"GOOD NIGHT."
CURES LIKE MAGIC
ALL ACHES & PAINS
SOLD BY THE AGENT
WHO PRESENTS YOU WITH THIS CHROMO.
SEE OTHER SIDE.

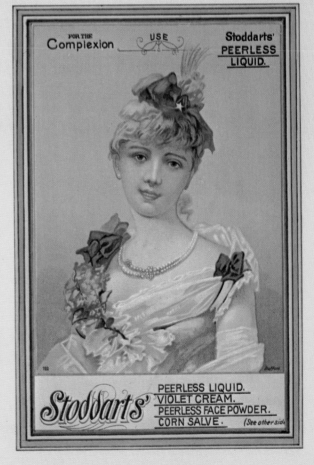

FOR THE
Complexion   USE   Stoddarts'
PEERLESS
LIQUID.

Stoddarts'   PEERLESS LIQUID.
VIOLET CREAM.
PEERLESS FACE POWDER.
CORN SALVE.   (See other side)

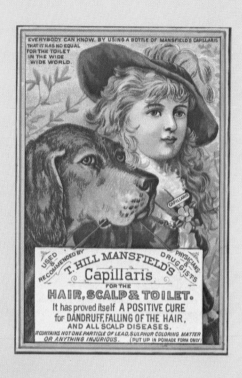

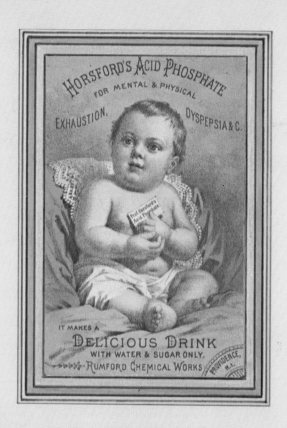

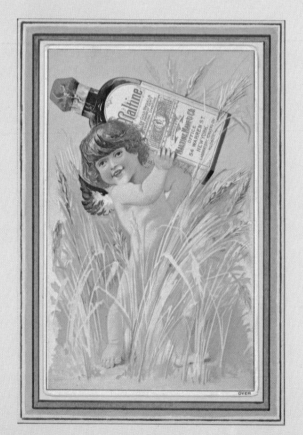

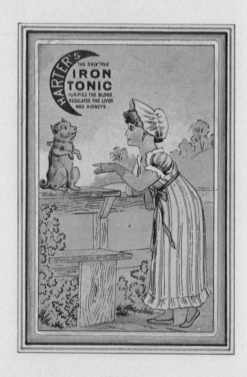

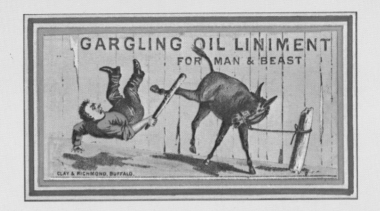

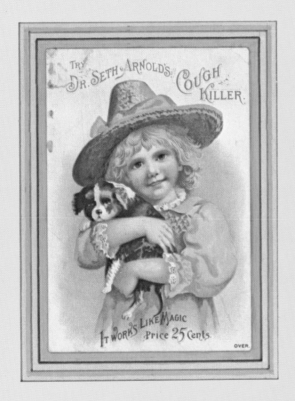

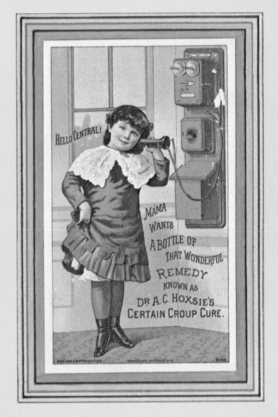

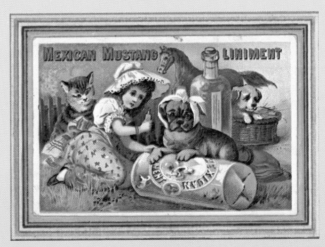

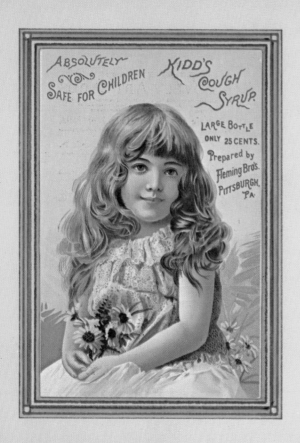

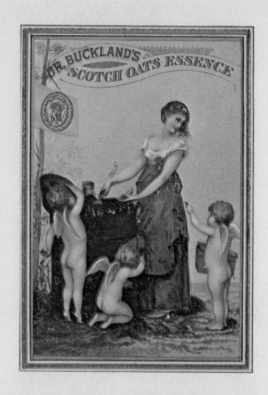

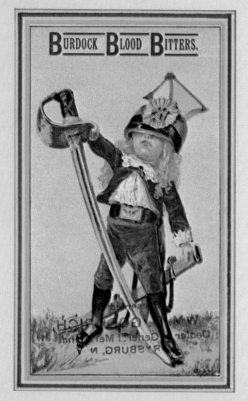

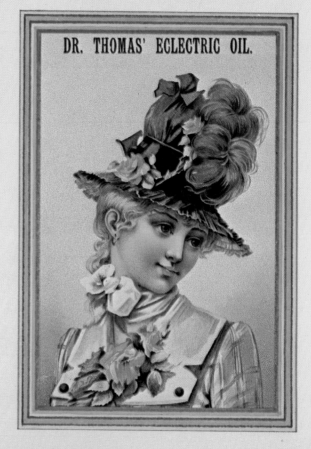

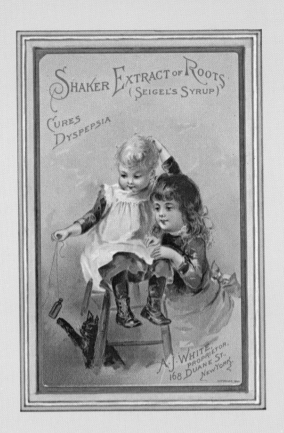

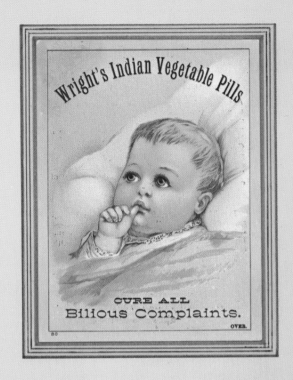

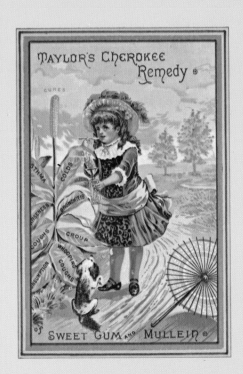

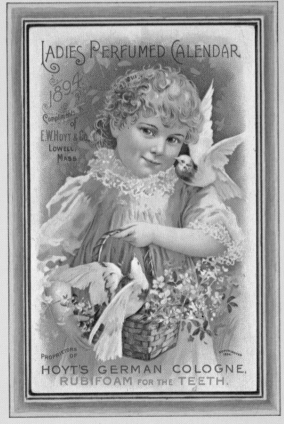

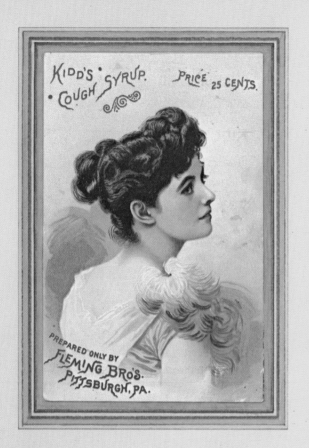

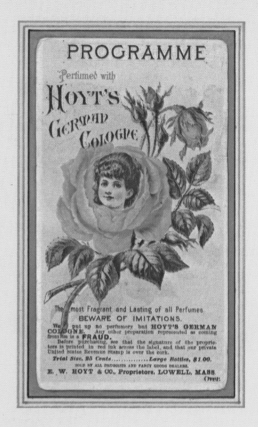

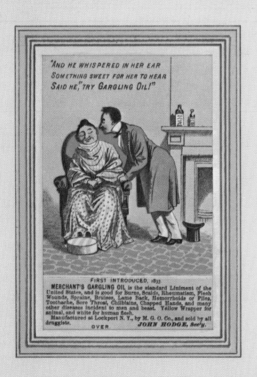

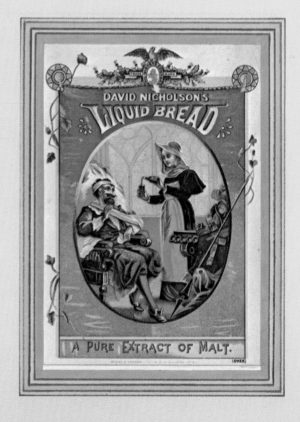

hinted, he had suffered untold agonies at the hands of white doctors whose greed and ignorance made life difficult for the dedicated Indian physician: "Dr. N's healing skill is original, having come down from many generations. Should Physicians speak evil of the Doctor's practice, pay no attention to what they say, for in so doing they speak evil of what they do not understand. What does the white man know of the Original Indian practice as it existed 400 years ago, and as it now exists? They know but little."

Dr. Newall's competition in the Indian pitch field included such colorful specimens as Dr. Vernett of Lockport, New York, who advertised himself as the "Mexican Indian Clarivoyant [sic]; the Seventh Son of the Seventh Son," and Dr. Green, the Indian Physician of Boston, whose medicines "are all VEGE-TABLE, and act in harmony with the laws of life; and so perfectly do they cleanse the blood of all disease, that out of several thousand cases of CANCER and SCROFULA which he has cured, not a case can be found where the disease has ever troubled them afterwards."[3] Dr. Newall was righteously con-

Sample Indian remedy trade card. WILLIAM H. HELFAND COLLECTION.

temptuous of such quacks. "They advertise largely what they can do," said the doctor, "and put on the Indian name; but when called upon for a trial, it is found they are different from the genuine Indian Doctor, and that their seeming knowledge is nothing but false pretension."

Two or three medicine workers would sometimes temporarily pool their talents and their money to create a tiny Indian show. The results were often ludicrous. In 1880 Donald McKay, a more or less genuine frontier character, joined a tiny company created by one of the several showmen who had adopted the name of the late Kit Carson. With the fake Carson was an Indian doctor named Red Fin, who was involved in the performance. Carson and Red Fin were an unscrupulous but affluent pair, a fact not lost on McKay, who was not strong on spelling and punctuation, but possessed a highly developed eye for the main chance. In a letter to his brother William, McKay described his adventures with the two showmen. "I came to Chicago," McKay wrote, "and thear I Met Kit Carson and a Man name of Red Fin. With Long hair and Pases himself For an indin Doctor him and Carson Made Lots of Money this Fall But you Know what Kind of a Dr he is he is a humbug But thay ar the ones that Makes the Money."[4] Carson and Red Fin hired McKay as a lecturer for twenty-five dollars a week, and the three moved on to Terre Haute, where McKay sent for his family. For ten days their show did good business. "But you Know how sum Men is," McKay added, "thay can't Presheat a good thing last night our long hair Dr had to git drunk and Raze hell and sum Fellow gave him a Belt on the nose and laid the indin Doctor Flat on the Floor With his long hair all over his Fase and this Morning thair Was a long Peas in the Paper . . . Kit has Bad luck With his indin Doctors he had a Man name Dr yella Stone and he Ran away With Carson dimond pin that cost Five Hundred and Fifty Dollars . . . I half to quit I am litel Excited our indin Doctor has chalang his Man to fait a dul and I Must go and see alltho I think thear Will be More Shit then Blood."

The fight and the attendant bad publicity had caused a rift between Carson and Red Fin, and at Carson's insistence the team was about to split up, although McKay was to begin working with the show again as soon as a replacement could be found for the Indian doctor. In spite of his temporary lay-off, McKay continued enthusiastic about the opportunities for easy money to be made with Carson, and he painted an attractive picture of the possibilities for his brother William, an Oregon doctor whom Carson wanted to hire. "I always tell the Peopel that I git all the Medicine From you I tell them that you git the old Women to gather the ruts and dry it and you send it to Me and thay think it is so." If William were to join Carson, McKay wrote, "I think you soon hav a Fortan For thar is no one on the Road this day that cin Beet Kit Carson to lecter on the street and advertiz. What he Wants With you is to go to Boston and open an indin Laboratory or an indin Arb Store . . . I think thear is Money in it him and yalla Ston Made Four thousand Dollars in three Weeks time I Would Bet My life that if you and him Was traveling that you could Make Hundred Dollars a day the year Round I dont tell you this to git you to cum But I only Michen this [to] see What Money cin be Made I only Wish that I was you For one year I would Know What to do With if I only had the nurve to do office Business I could Parliz the Peopel But I cant lie to them When thay set clos to Me But out on the streets I cin tell More lise then Patch hell a Mile." William, who grew interested in the possibility of an alliance with Carson, wrote to Buffalo Bill Cody for advice and received a brief and clear-eyed assessment of the showman. "If I was a regular doctor in the U.S.A. I would not give it up and take chances on an outside speculation," Cody wrote. "Kit Carson is a smart fellow, but how responsible I won't say."[5]

Indian show operators like Carson placed a premium on flamboyance: most were walking advertisements for their shows, dressing in some exotic variation of Indian or frontier dress. Carson himself had sported the stolen five-hundred-and-fifty-dollar diamond pin; and in 1888, when a man's suit of good quality could be purchased for fifteen dollars or less, Donald McKay's new employer, Colonel T. A. Edwards of the Oregon Indian Medicine Company, provided his star attraction with a forty-dollar suit and a sixteen-dollar hat—probably the first of a line of spectacular buckskin outfits in which

McKay was pictured on Oregon labels and in the company's publications.[6] Dr. Lamereux, "the world-renowned Indian fighter, scout and medicine man," appeared dressed from head to toe in black velvet, with twenty-dollar gold pieces for coat buttons and ten-dollar gold pieces for buttons on his vest. His shoulder-length black hair was topped by a huge sombrero around which a lariat used in his performance was coiled.[7] Captain Jim Brown favored a more cheerful outfit. "He had on a pair of long corduroy pants stuffed into black boots with red bands and a star in their tops," wrote a spectator at Captain Jim's show. "His shirt was blue silk without the collar buttoned, and a big red handkerchief went under the collar and was tied down on his chest. . . . His hat was white and big with a wide brim. . . . He had a big diamond ring on each one of his hands. His belt was wide and buckled with gold stars."[8]

Perhaps the ultimate frontier fantasy was the costume created by Nevada Ned Oliver in 1886, when he operated his own show, Nevada Ned's Big Indian Village. "While playing the Horseshoe in Jersey City earlier in 1886," Oliver wrote, "I had added ten-dollar gold pieces as buttons on my velvet and corduroy jackets, five-dollar gold coins as buttons on my fancy vests, three-dollar gold pieces as cuff links. Around my neck I wore a chain of half eagles, meeting in a fifty-dollar gold slug and extending on to the watch pocket and a watch that weighed a pound. . . . To relieve this Quakerish simplicity, I wore $3,000 worth of real diamonds and two gold-mounted .44's. My mustache was long and prettily waxed to points, my clothes foppish in the extreme. In such fashion I liked to stroll up Broadway or through the markets in Washington and Fulton streets, followed by bootblacks, newsboys and messengers, who could not decide whether to hoot or cheer."[9] It was all the same to Oliver for whom—as for all medicine showmen—the only real calamity lay in not being noticed at all.

The big Indian shows like Nevada Ned's provided fairly substantial entertainment in the manner of the Healy and Bigelow units. Dr. James M. Solomon (who claimed to be a lineal descendant of King Philip, sachem of the Wampanoags, as well as the seventh son of old Dr. Solomon, the great root and

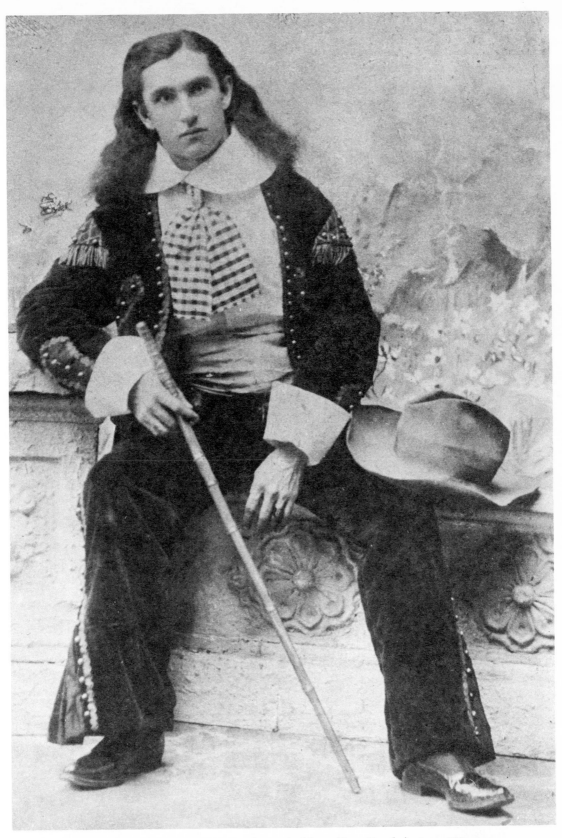

A medicine showman, Joseph F. Golden (Joe Steele), in a Western outfit.　MUSEUM OF THE CITY OF NEW YORK.

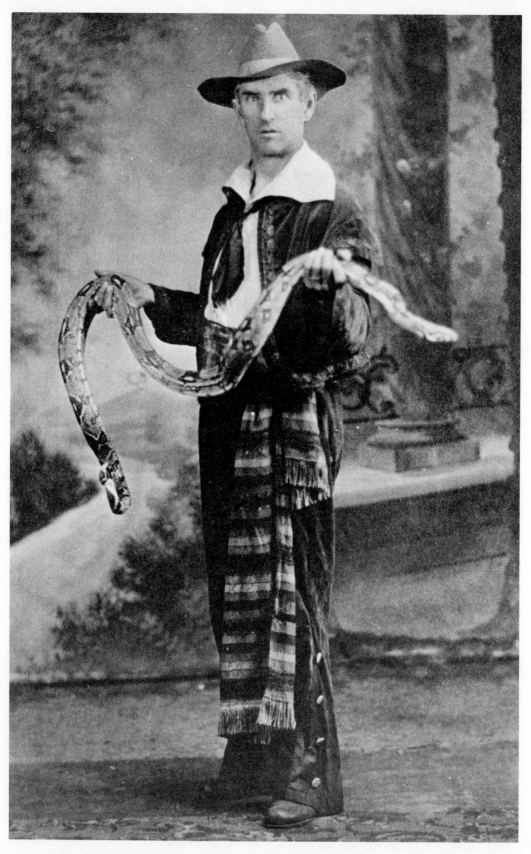

Joseph F. Golden in later years. MUSEUM OF THE CITY OF NEW YORK.

herb doctor of Attleboro, Massachusetts) drew audiences to his traveling Indian Wigwam with a "Genuine Band of Winnebago Indians" who presented "Indian Music, Marriage Ceremonies, Going to Battle, &c., Assisted by a Troupe of First-Class Comedians, and Mr. T. F. Hayes, Lecturer on Medicine."[10] Shows of this sort began with a march down the aisles by the Indians to the tune of "The Star-Spangled Banner" and a war dance followed by a one-act comedy, a minstrel routine, or a high-kicking song and dance number for the men and an exotic mind-reading act designed to please the ladies.[11]

Small companies gave only a simple show, usually nothing more than a few songs and banjo solos, along with some jokes and magic tricks or bits of ventriloquism. In Harry Leon Wilson's novel *Professor, How Could You!* a tiny show featured a lecturer who doubled as entertainer, and a fake Indian—a college professor who had abandoned teaching for the romance of the road. The performance started with a song by Jackson, the lecturer-entertainer, "a rollicking and noisy ballad in the negro dialect in which the vocalist was required to laugh heartily midway in the chorus."[12] The song drew a crowd and Jackson launched into a ventriloquist's act: clutching a Negro dummy in one hand and an Irish dummy in the other, he began a series of hoary dialect jokes designed to soften up the crowd for his Indian pitch. After they had warmed to the performance, Jackson began a stock Indian show story, the tale of how he had saved the life of a famous Indian chief who, in grateful appreciation, gave him the secret of a miraculous medicine composed of life-giving roots and herbs.[13]

There were dozens of variations on the stock "snatched from the jaws of death" story, in which the lecturer saved the life of an Indian or, like Texas Charlie Bigelow, had his own life saved by some miracle of Indian pharmacology. With a passion for dime novel melodrama, both patent medicine almanacs and medicine show lecturers recounted sensational tales of the origins of their cure-alls. Indian Blood Syrup provided customers with a saga entitled *Captured and Branded by the Camanche* [sic] *Indians in the Year 1860,* and Judson's Mountain Herb Pills issued *The Rescue of Tula* in which Dr. Cunard, the hero, saves an Aztec princess from death at the stake

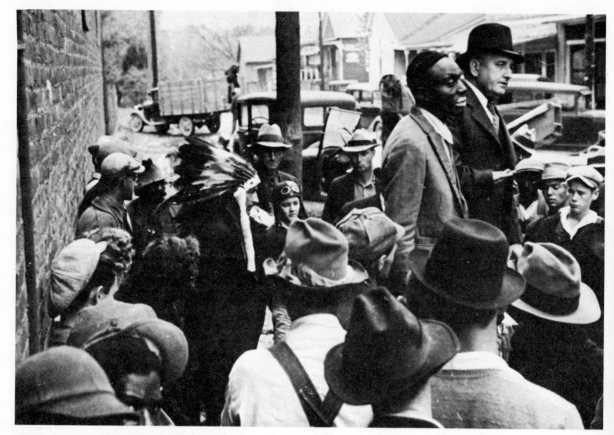

Small street-corner medicine show with an Indian and a Jake character, Huntingdon, Tennessee, 1935.

PHOTO BY SHAHN. LIBRARY OF CONGRESS.

and is rewarded with the secret of Mountain Herb Pills.[14] Captain Jim Brown combined the usual stories in his medicine lecture. He claimed to have been lost in a snowstorm and would have died if he had not been found by an old Indian whose life he had once saved. The Indian took Captain Jim to his village, where the white man's strength was restored by a secret remedy brewed by the tribe's medicine man. As he regained his health, Captain Jim became interested in the medicine's secret, which the Indians refused to divulge. Unlike the Kickapoos, they had not had the foresight to create a medicine that defied chemical analysis and, for the sake of suffering white humanity, Captain Jim spirited away some of the potion to a chemist who was able to reveal its secret.[15]

After the account of the medicine's mysterious origins, an Indian or an Indian impersonator was often produced as its creator and asked to say a few words in his native tongue to the assembled crowd: Wilson's professor-turned-Indian chanted a Vedic hymn; Dr. Snodgrass of Robert Lewis Taylor's *Journey to Matecumbe*, who claimed to have been adopted by the Indians, muttered nonsense syllables that more or less passed for Choctaw; and Nevada Ned Oliver offered audiences stirring on-the-spot translations of Indian orations of which he could not understand a word.[16] Next came the sale, along with a ritualized sales pitch and, in some cases, free diagnosis on-stage.[17] A number of operators paved the way for their pitches with testimonials from the crowd.[18] Sometimes these were earnest statements from people who genuinely believed they had been cured by the showman's remedies; often, however, the testimonials came from members of the company pretending to be spectators, or from locals who were willing to endorse anything for a fee. In either case the effect was the same—the beginnings of the kind of mass anxiety that made the audience accept the lecturer's medicine pitch at face value. One especially shrewd operator passed out his medicine before he commenced his pitch, asking spectators to clutch the lifesaving bottles as he described in detail the symptoms of the hideous diseases cured by his Indian panacea.[19]

The heart of the stock Indian medicine sales pitch was the same natural cure idea favored by patent medicine promoters of all sorts since the eighteenth century. Indians were healthier than whites, the lecturer pointed out, and the reason lay in the secret remedy about to be dispensed:

> Ladies and Gentlemen! Some good folks devote their lives to saving souls; others in accumulating wealth. I am here this evening, not only to entertain you, but to relieve suffering humanity of its aches and pains. I call your attention to the bottle I hold in my hand, containing one of the greatest gifts to man. This famous Indian Herb Medicine is made from a formula handed down from generation to generation by my forefathers, who were chiefs of the Osage Indians. Did you ever hear of an Osage Indian having rheu-

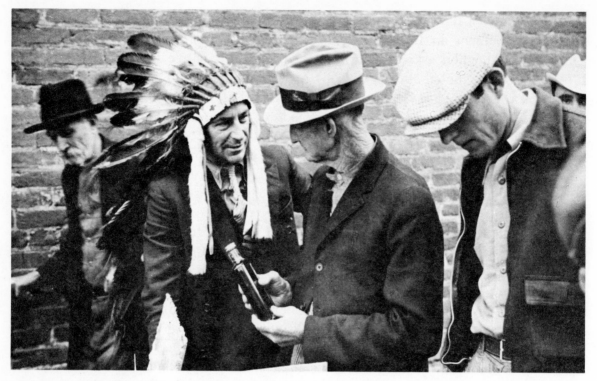

Medicine show Indian selling tonic, Huntingdon, Tennessee, 1935.
LIBRARY OF CONGRESS.

matism? No! Ladies and gentlemen! Did you ever
hear of an Osage Indian having scarlet fever, sore
throat or colds? A thousand times, no! It is written in
the white man's Bible that three score and ten is a long
life, but it is a common occurrence for an Osage Indian to live to be a hundred years old and never suffer
a pain or an ache. How does he accomplish this wonderful feat? He does it with the aid of this wonderful
medicine I now hold before you. The Indian gave you
America and now he gives you the magic secret of
health and happiness with long life, the greatest blessing of all.[20]

The sales pitch, reinforced by a money-back guarantee and
featuring special, ridiculously low prices designed to introduce
the product to new sufferers, continued until the lecturer
felt that the audience was his. Then the banjos struck up a tune

Old Indian Liver and Kidney Tonic

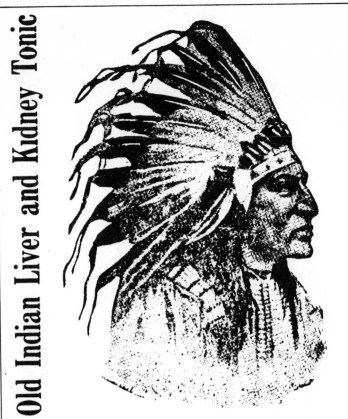

The Unfailing Remedy for Laziness and a Drowsy, Tired, Sleepy Feeling

It takes the place of Calomel without any restriction of habit or diet while taking. It positively will not make you sick, gripe or nauseate you in the slightest way like Calomel Pills and most all the various kinds of liquid liver medicines. There are very few people in this world today who feel so well that a few doses of this medicine would not make them feel a great deal better and give them a new lease on life.

It makes the eye bright, clears up the complexion, quickens the senses and is a most wonderful tonic and appetizer.

Relieves a bad cold or cough in one day.

Relieves la grippe in one day.

Relieves fever in one day.

Relieves weakness and tired feeling in one day.

Relieves pain in the neck, side, shoulder, back or hips in one day . Relieves bad headache in two hours.

Relieves sick stomach, belching, gas on stomach in three hours.

Relieves the worst case of drunkenness in six hours.

Relieves bladder and kidney trouble.

Relieves rheumatism, giving quick relief from the pain.

Relieves female diseases and women's troubles.

Five or six doses will fix you so your work will not tire you one particle and you can do your work with ten times the ease.

It will work three to four gallons of bile from the system that is as black as any ink that you ever saw come out of any ink bottle. We will pay One Hundred Dollars Reward if it gripes a particle or makes you sick in the slightest way.

(Your name as manufacturer printed here in this space.)

Sample Indian remedy advertisement.

and all of the spare performers took to the aisles for the first sale of the evening.

"All of this time," wrote an observer at an Indian show, "the Indians kept chanting monotonously and beating their tom-toms, the doctor himself roaring like a bull, while the min-strels kept up a furious ragtime dancing until the sweat rolled down their black faces."[21] In most companies salesmen were given only one or two bottles each time they dashed to the stage to replenish their supply of medicine. The air was filled with the cry, "All sold out, Doctor!" and spectators, caught up in the noise and excitement, were convinced that hundreds of bottles were sold for every dozen that actually changed hands.[22] After the sale, little troupes would continue for as long as they could hold a crowd with a combination of pitches, giveaways, banjo music, and vocal renderings of the senti-mental favorites of the day.[23] Larger shows proceeded through more Indian dances and minstrel and vaudeville acts, with perhaps two more sales before the afterpiece, the tradi-tional final act of the medicine show.

Like other showmen, owners of many of the independent Indian shows simply mixed their own remedies in hotel bath-tubs, buying the bottles and labels wherever possible and the ingredients from local druggists or drug wholesalers.[24] Others ordered standard remedies which were provided with their own personal labels by the supply house: the makers of Old Indian Liver and Kidney Tonic, for example, distributed sam-ple advertising cards to medicine men with the suggestion that the showman's name could be inserted on the card as the manufacturer of the concoction, somewhat vaguely described as an unfailing remedy for "Laziness and a Drowsy, Tired, Sleepy Feeling."[25] Still other medicine men acted as agents for one of the lines of Indian products prepared by such whole-salers as the Suter Remedy Company, which provided show-men with Dr. Ranell's Indian Herb Tablets, Pain-Expeller and Rattle Snake Oil, and Indian Corn Remover, Worm Eradicator, and Tape-Worm Expeller.[26] By far the most important supplier of Indian remedies to independents, however, was the Oregon Indian Medicine Company of Corry, Pennsylvania, creators of Ka-Ton-Ka, "The Only Indian Medicine on Earth Backed with BANKABLE Paper."[27]

8

OREGON

Of course, the *Grafter*, the *Slum Slinger*, the
Fakir, will always exist, after their fashion—
and be broke seven eights of the time. The
Legitimate Lecturer and Manager will still go
on his way *Making Money*.

Oregon Indian Medicine Company brochure

The Oregon Indian Medicine Company was the creation of
Colonel T. A. Edwards, a colorful frontier character and
former circus manager.[1] Edwards was born in Saugerties, New
York, in 1832. As a child he was bound out to a farmer from
whom he ran away to sea, serving first as a cabin boy on an
ocean liner and then as a sailor on a whaling vessel. After his
return to the United States, he worked for a time as business
manager for the Spaulding and Rogers Circus and later for the
John Robinson Circus. In 1857 Edwards joined the expedition
against the Mormons under the command of General Albert
Sidney Johnston, and in the two years that followed was involved in the gold rush at Pike's Peak. After a dull interlude as
an employee of the Memphis Transportation Company, Edwards joined the secret service at the outbreak of the Civil
War and served for several years as a spy behind Confederate
lines.[2] In 1864 he became a scout for General Steele in Arkansas, and after the war continued his career as both spy and
scout under General Cooke in the Oregon territory.

"HEALTH OR MONEY RESTORED."
Col. T. A. EDWARDS.

At one day's sight pay to the

Order of _____ $ 1⁰⁰⁄₁₀₀

One _____ ⁰⁰⁄₁₀₀ *Dollars,*

Value received and charge the same to account of

To CITIZENS' NATIONAL BANK, | *Oregon Indian Med. Co.*
CORRY, PA.

189___ No.___

The Only Indian Medicine on Earth
Backed with BANKABLE Paper.

$100 REWARD If the above Draft is not as GOOD AS GOLD at said Bank for ONE DOLLAR when issued with A BOTTLE OF KA-TON-KA for the cure of Diseases of Liver, Kidneys, Stomach and Blood

We Have a cure for the People. We have a System of guaranteeing a CURE.

A DRAFT WITH EVERY BOTTLE

Our Customers cannot Lose their MONEY if we Fail to CURE.

Is there a Physician in your City who will give you his Check or Draft on his Bank or your money back if he fails to cure You?

KA-TON-KA

is the Original Indian Medicine derived from the Indians. Beware of the many imitations, substitutes and impostors.

The Oregon INDIAN Medicine Co.

is the Only Indian Medicine Co. that backs up its Cures with BANKABLE PAPER.

"THEIR MEDICINES CURE"

Circular, Oregon Indian Medicine Company.

It was in Oregon that Edwards first came across the flamboyant Donald McKay. McKay, a trapper and trader, had been born in 1836, the son of a white man and an Indian woman.[3] Ironically, McKay was disliked and distrusted by the Indians with whom his name came to be linked, although he had the confidence of white army officers who used him as a scout and interpreter. In 1873 he was hired by the Army to accompany a band of Indians from the Warm Spring Reservation in Oregon in what was to become a famous incident in the Modoc War. The scouts were sent to track down the rebel Modoc leader, Captain Jack, in the craters and caverns of the barren California Lava Beds. Captain Jack was found, and, after a desperate fight, he and his warriors were forced to scatter. At length, starving and exhausted, Captain Jack surrendered and was tried and executed. The spectacular ending of the Modoc War made headlines in Eastern newspapers. Within a short time showmen, sensing potentially profitable Western attractions, began to take over: the body of Captain Jack was stolen from its grave, embalmed, and toured as a carnival attraction in the East, and Edwards, recalling his circus training, took the Warm Springs scouts to Europe in 1874 and to the Philadelphia Centennial Exhibition of 1876 as glorified sideshow attractions.[4]

The Indians and McKay shortly became the promotional hook on which Edwards hung his next venture, the Oregon Indian Medicine Company, organized in Pittsburgh in 1876. Edwards's advertising strongly implied that Ka-Ton-Ka, his principal cure-all, and the rest of the Oregon products, were manufactured by McKay and the Indians of the Umatilla Reservation in Oregon.[5] In fact, the medicines were made in Pittsburgh and later in Corry, Pennsylvania, where the company moved in the mid-eighties. Edwards did flirt briefly with the idea of actually opening an Oregon plant under the supervision of McKay's brother, but he abandoned it because of the difficulty of getting bottles blown in the West.[6] The fiction that Oregon remedies were actually concocted by the Indians themselves in the depths of the forest—an idea shortly borrowed by Healy and Bigelow—had a strong appeal from the

first, and Edwards built up a prosperous medicine show operation with a small laboratory and a number of advertising units
traveling throughout the East and the Midwest, as well as a
growing wholesale business. "I hav only Bean here two days,"
wrote McKay on a visit to Corry in 1888, "and thar Was over
two thousand Dollars orders Was sent for from Difrent Druges
Stors from Difrent Parts of this state so you Cin see how the
Ka ton Ka is seling."[7] At the plant, McKay found six people
employed full-time bottling Oregon remedies; and he assured
his brother that the Colonel "Will Be a Rich Man in a few
years."[8] By 1892 Edwards owned valuable property in Corry
and was toying with the idea of retiring to California; by 1896
he claimed to have thirty-seven advertising units on the
road.[9]

The returns were excellent, but it was risky to operate a
string of traveling units. McKay, whose job it was to supervise
the road companies, wrote of the vicissitudes of medicine show
business: "it has bin snow and raining the streets are all Full of
Watter & Mud & sluch Busniss is not good at Present For this
theatre has Bin a lagar Beer so you see how it is."[10] A string of
bad houses or a long siege of wet weather could eat up profits
with incredible swiftness when a full medicine show company
of ten or a dozen had to be paid each week in spite of poor
business or no business at all. "You dont Know," McKay told
his brother, "how Much it takes to advertise."[11] Before the
turn of the century Edwards turned increasingly toward the
safer wholesale medicine business, merely furnishing independent showmen with drugs and the ubiquitous "paper" that
made it possible for a troupe to suggest that it was an official
Oregon Indian Medicine Company unit. In *The Billboard* and
other publications read by pitchmen and medicine showmen,
the company inserted advertisements, often with pictures of
Donald McKay in his picturesque frontier outfits, inviting "Independent Managers and Doctors" to handle the Oregon
line.[12]

The advertisements and flyers offered tantalizing proposi-
tions to every sort of showman and peddler. "Lady Canvass-
ers" were advised that they could make as much as forty dollars a week selling Oregon products door to door, while men

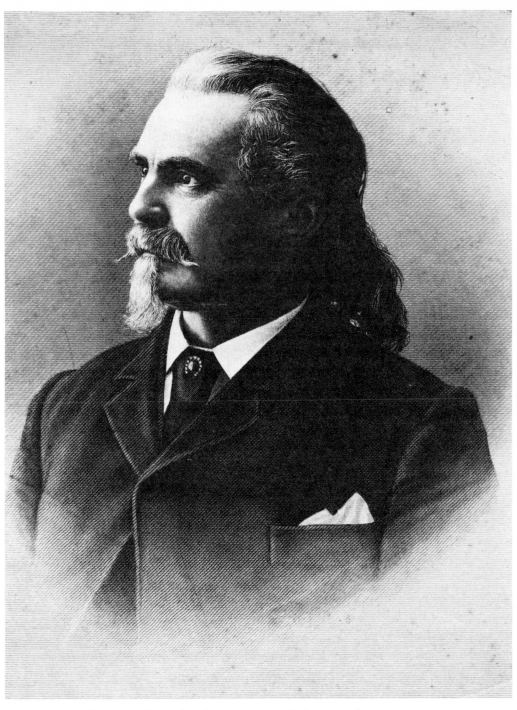

Colonel T. A. Edwards of the Oregon Indian Medicine Company.

who possessed a horse and buggy were assured that they could earn more in a year driving through the countryside than a storekeeper with $15,000 worth of stock behind the counter. Men who could muster the elements of a small show like those sent out by the Hamlin Wizard Oil Company (a team, a fancy wagon, a parlor organ, and some musicians and singers) were almost certain, the advertisements said, to take in at least $2,-000 each year and perhaps as much as $6,000.[13]

In 1890 the Oregon products included Indian Ka-Ton-Ka, in both liquid and powdered form, Nez Percé Catarrh Snuff, Indian Cough Syrup, Modoc Oil, War Paint Ointment, Warm Springs Consumption Cure, and Donald McKay's Indian Worm Eradicator.[14] A former Oregon employee described the manufacture of the tapeworm pills. "There was a fine kind of flimsy tissue paper we bought," he said. "I cut it into narrow strips like carpet rags. Then I would roll a strip up tightly and carefully make an egg shaped pill. It was then dipped in a syrup that would be quite hard when dried. The pills would stand quite a lot of rattling around in a box without the coating peeling off."[15] The coating of course disappeared in the human digestive tract, and the long roll of tissue paper became convincing evidence of the tapeworm's demise and the efficacy of Indian Worm Eradicator. Later, Edwards added a number of new items to tempt showmen, including Ka-Ton-Ka pills, Wasco Cough Drops, Quillaia Soap, Mox-ci-tong, and Woman's Friend.[16] Ka-Ton-Ka, in its various forms, like Healy and Bigelow's Sagwa, was the staple item, an essentially innocuous but invigorating stomachic, largely made up of sugar, aloes, and baking soda, and containing a hefty 20 percent alcohol.[17] In private, Edwards was disarmingly objective about the merits of Ka-Ton-Ka. He was once asked whether he took the tonic himself. "That ain't to take," he is supposed to have replied. "It's made to sell."[18]

It sold amazingly well and—at least in theory—provided a Ka-Ton-Ka showman with an enormous profit on a relatively small initial investment. In the last years of the nineteenth century, for example, Edwards sold bottled Ka-Ton-Ka to independent showmen for $2.00 a dozen, and the powdered variety for $1.00 per dozen boxes. The same remedies were sold by the showmen to druggists in the towns where they played for $7.50 and $3.50 a dozen respectively. The price to spectators at the shows was suggested by Edwards to be $1.00 each for the bottled remedy and fifty cents each for the powder—or, in most cases, whatever traffic would bear since Edwards refused to supply showmen who were known to cut prices but not those who raised them when the opportunity arose.[19]

As a unique incentive to handle Oregon products, Edwards allowed dealers to issue a money-back guarantee with every bottle of Ka-Ton-Ka. In the nineties, the guarantee, a draft for one dollar on the Citizen's National Bank of Corry, was accompanied by so much complicated rhetoric that it was almost impossible to determine whether the company was offering one dollar or one hundred in case Ka-Ton-Ka failed to do its work —or, for that matter, how one qualified for a refund in the first place.[20] After 1910, probably because of the increasingly close watch being kept on patent medicine men by the government, the company tamed the language of the guarantee somewhat and added a relatively clear description of how the dissatisfied user obtained his money. But the apparent clarity of the guarantee masked a nightmare of complications: after taking Ka-Ton-Ka for three months, according to directions, for a disease for which it was recommended, and using no other remedies or stimulants during that time, the uncured sufferer was entitled to begin the process of dunning Oregon. He was first required to send all the empty bottles he had purchased back to the company headquarters prepaid. Next he was asked to fill out a form certifying that he had purchased the bottles, listing the date on which each was purchased and the name of the agent. Having completed this form, he had only to go to a notary public and obtain his signature and seal along with the signatures of three additional reliable witnesses. Then he was required to send the form to the Corry National Bank. When the bottles had been received at company headquarters and the properly completed form was in the hands of the bank, the ailing one—probably now in a serious decline because of the exertion—was awarded his money. Presumably he was expecting a dollar for each bottle he had taken during his unsuccessful three months' cure, a sum that might at least have reimbursed him for postage and the notary's fee, and provided something for his trouble. But the bank draft on the rear of the form was for a single dollar. In fact, he would have had to fill out a new form and have it witnessed and notarized for each bottle on which he hoped to collect—a technicality of which the company would no doubt have been pleased to inform him at the completion of the obstacle course.[21]

Edwards also supplied showmen with a complete line of free Oregon paper, including packets containing two different three-sheet lithographs, eight different one-sheets, and ten assorted half-sheet lithographs, along with a dozen plainer one-sheet posters. With these came a line of "small paper"—mostly flyers to be distributed to the audience at the show—and a miscellaneous selection of admission tickets, present tickets, and contest ballots. With each bottle of Ka-Ton-Ka purchased by the showman, Edwards also sent a novelty calendar or a copy of a pamphlet supposedly written by Donald McKay called *Indian Scout Life*, which could be given away as premiums by the showman.[22]

Indian Scout Life is in the tradition of the *Kickapoo Indian Magazine* and other Healy and Bigelow publications, with a heavy dose of house advertisements and testimonials, and filler extracted from other patent medicine almanacs and fact books. The main attraction of *Indian Scout Life* is a florid biographical sketch of McKay which traces his career as guide, scout, interpreter, and Indian fighter through the usual sort of sanguinary frontier anecdotes—McKay shot through both hips, struck by lightning, wounded by a poisoned arrow, and so on. For those who craved more of McKay's Western adventures, an advertisement in *Indian Scout Life* announced a longer work, *Daring Donald McKay, or the Last War-Trail of the Modocs*, which could be obtained from Oregon Indian Medicine dealers or directly from Colonel Edwards in Corry.[23] Like Texas Charlie Bigelow of Kickapoo, Donald McKay was an official company hero who admitted to no rivals as a professional Westerner. "The record that stands behind Donald McKay stamps him as the greatest Indian fighter and government scout that ever lived," said *Indian Scout Life*. "The numerous dime novel heroes, long-haired stage strutters, and

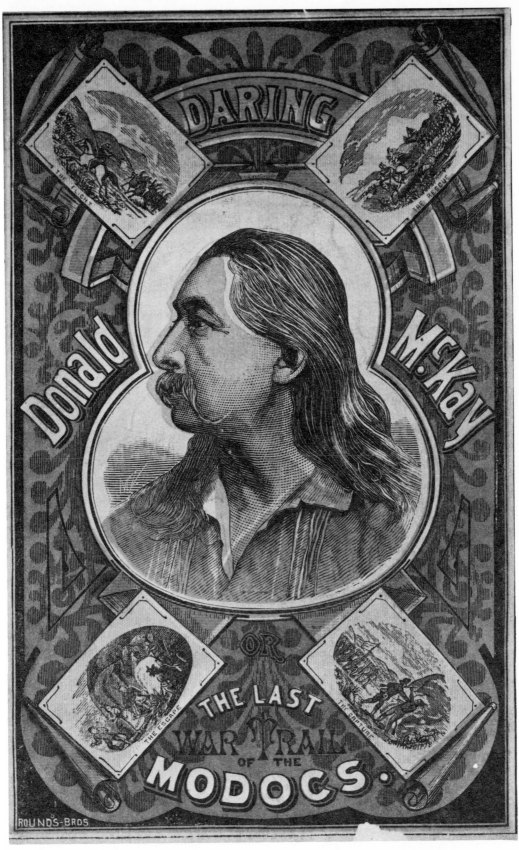

Cover of *Daring Donald McKay, or the Last War-Trail of the Mo-docs.*

Wild West exponents, who receive their plaudits from large audiences of our modern civilization, are but poor imitators of a life spent in actual service by an Indian whose experience with danger would make those parlor entertainers and ex-cow-punchers wish to be excused."[24]

As the new century progressed, it all made very little difference—the public was no longer really interested. McKay died in 1894 and Colonel Edwards in 1904. After the colonel's death, the company passed to his daughter, a Mrs. Van Vleck, who ran it for a time to increasingly dwindling profits, ultimately abandoning the Indian image and changing the name of her line to Modern Miracles.[25] The Indian medicine show boom was over. The Indian show gradually gave way to a less exotic kind of vaudeville performance.[26] T. P. Kelley, a Canadian medicine man with a large vaudeville show, dismissed his Indian competitors as already insignificant in the late nineties. Although Kickapoo units played ahead of Kelley in the Maritime Provinces, he claimed that they had ceased to be formidable competition. The public, said Kelley, had "grown weary of their painted faces, war dances, waving tomahawks, and their guttural promises of 'Medicine heap good.'"[27] Like the Wild West show, the Indian medicine show faded and declined in the twentieth century, in large part the victim of the Western film, which presented realistic and spectacular Western adventures that could never be duplicated with live performers on the road.

A few Indian pitchmen and small independent Indian companies lasted into the thirties in spite of increasing competition from the straight variety medicine shows.[28] In 1929 Nevada Ned Oliver recalled a dozen or more Indian showmen who were still on the road, and as late as 1936 it was still possible to see performances by the Old-Fashioned Indian Medicine Company, the Blackhawk Medicine Company, the Indian Medicine Company Show, the Winona Medicine Company of the Sioux Tribe, the Pawnee Indian Remedy Company, the Choctaw Indian Medicine Show, the Kiowa Indian Medicine and Vaudeville Company, and the Iroquois Famous Indian Remedies Company of Harlem.[29] But such companies were anomalies. The real end of the Indian show had come long before with the decline and fall of Healy and Bigelow's famous Kickapoo Indian Medicine Company.

Sometime during the nineties Healy sold out to Bigelow and moved to Australia. Texas Charlie Bigelow held out until 1912 when, like his former partner, he went in search of greener pastures.[30] Moving to England, Bigelow began to manufacture a line of remedies identical to the old Kickapoo products, calling his most popular tonic Kimco in honor of the Kickapoo Indian Medicine Company. Later, with Arthur Healy, one of John Healy's sons, Texas Charlie planned a chain of painless dental parlors in Great Britain. The chain never materialized, although the basic idea was to be used with spectacular success in the United States by the ex-Kickapoo Indian agent, Dr. Painless Parker.[31] Texas Charlie died during World War I.[32]

Letter to a medicine showman.   WILLIAM H. HELFAND COLLECTION.

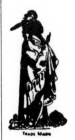

Removed to 639 N. Broad Street, Philadelphia, Pa.

OFFICE OF

THE KICKAPOO INDIAN MEDICINE CO. INC.

FORMERLY NEW HAVEN, CONN.

CLINTONVILLE, CONN.

Phila. Dec. 23rd,   1914.

Dr. W. H. Kelley,
117 Standart St.,
Syracuse, N. Y.

Dear Doctor:

As we discontinued the pratice of advertising through traveling shows, we are unable to accept your proposition.

yours truly,

EP/AET   THE KICKAPOO INDIAN MED. CO.

The firm to which he sold the Kickapoo Indian Medicine Company had very different promotional ideas from those of Healy and Bigelow, and although Kickapoo Indian Sagwa continued to sell well in country drugstores and general stores into the twenties, as early as 1914 the company was tersely advising showmen that it was out of the medicine show business for good.[33]

Not long after Texas Charlie's death, a nostalgic article appeared in the New Haven *Register*. "Is there any likelihood," asked the correspondent, "of our ever seeing again anything like the war dances and the fine horses and the feathered big medicine men and the comely young squaws, and the trick shooting and the fine basket work and the up-to-date cracks and quips of the street salesman who went with the Kickapoo Indian show? And the snappy bands with the staccato urge, always staccato?"[34] The question was rhetorical; by the twenties the Indian medicine show was already a quaint half-forgotten curiosity.

UP IN ALL THE
ACTS AND BITS

Wanted, For the Ku-Ver-O Medicine Co.'s *Opera House Show,* all kinds of Medicine performers, who can make good for two weeks. Long engagement for right people. Kickers, Knockers, Boozers, and Managers save postage. Piano player to double on stage needed. Salary sure every Sunday morning; plenty of money behind this show, besides I always got the coin and do not close the year round. The three Everetts, the Hermans, Walter Ross and Billy Vandy, write. Address Dr. W. D. Moore, Corner of Oliver and Central Aves., Cincinnati, Ohio.

The Billboard advertisement

From the very beginning, variety acts had been a part of virtually all medicine shows. Most street workers introduced at least a few sleight-of-hand tricks, a comic monologue, or some banjo solos between their pitches; the Kickapoo shows of the eighties and nineties alternated vaudeville and circus acts with their war dances and mock powwows; and even the professionally pious Quaker Healers leavened their sermons with clog dances and minstrel routines. After the turn of the nineteenth century the character of the medicine show began to change.

Vaudeville dominated popular entertainment in the cities and towns, and in the rural areas medicine show companies began to place more emphasis on vaudeville acts and less on exotic atmosphere and costumes. The old-fashioned Indian, Oriental, and Quaker shows gradually gave way to a vaudeville performance interrupted by medicine lectures and sales. The twentieth-century medicine shows, however, were not simply small-time vaudeville with pauses for commercial messages. They developed their own unique brand of variety out of a curious mixture of vaudeville, burlesque, dime museum material, and the minstrel show.

Not all later medicine shows used a variety format. Some presented full-length plays or, more often, tabloid versions of plays, and a few companies carried a small circus or a burlesque show, although burlesque was usually considered too "strong" for the sort of small-town family audiences characteristically attracted by medicine show companies.[1] The dramatic fare presented by troupes carrying plays was not very different from the sort of thing featured by small tent repertoire companies—*The Drunkard, Ten Nights in a Barroom, Kathleen Mavourneen,* and standard "Toby and Suzy" pieces, featuring a carrot-topped rustic named Toby and a gangling country girl with a calico dress and pigtails, known as Suzy or "The Silly Kid."[2] It was a repertoire medicine show company that Sinclair Lewis described in *Main Street:*

> Carol attended the only professional play that came to Gopher Prairie that spring. It was a "tent show, presenting snappy new dramas under canvas." The hard-working actors doubled in brass, and took tickets; and between acts sang about the moon in June, and sold Dr. Wintergreen's Surefire Tonic for Ills of the Heart, Lungs, Kidneys, and Bowels. They presented "Sunbonnet Nell: A Dramatic Comedy of the Ozarks," with J. Witherbee Boothby wringing the soul by his resonant "Yuh ain't done right by mah little gal, Mr. City Man, but yer a-goin' to find that back in these-yere hills there's honest folks and good shots!"
> The audience, on planks beneath the patched tent, admired Mr. Boothby's beard and long rifle; stamped their feet in the dust at the spectacle of his heroism;

COMING!

German Medicine Company

IN HIGH CLASS

Vaudeville!

THE EVENT OF THE SEASON.

SPECIAL PROGRAME

New Acts, New Faces. New Features.

ONE CONTINOUS ROUND OF PLEASURE.

Sterling Specialtes,
   Dainty Dancers.
Clever Comedians,
   Sweet Singers,

An unrivalled array of bright and catchy AMUSEMENT.

Nothing like it ever presented ir your town by a Medicine Co.

Special attention is given to the comfort of LADIES and CHILDREN. Polite and attentive Ushers are always in attendance.

ADMISSION 10 CENTS.

Stock showbill, German Medicine Company.

shouted when the comedian aped the City Lady's use of a lorgnon by looking through a doughnut stuck on a fork; wept visibly over Mr. Boothby's Little Gal Nell, who was also Mr. Boothby's legal wife Pearl, and when the curtain went down, listened respectfully to Mr. Boothby's lecture on Dr. Wintergreen's tonic as a cure for tape-worms, which he illustrated by horrible pallid objects curled in a bottle of yellowing alcohol.[3]

On the whole, the sort of production described by Lewis, although it was featured by a few companies, never loomed very large in the world of the medicine show. Straight plays were probably avoided by most showmen because the majority were not willing to assume the risk of rehearsing a stock company only to have a performer leave or take sick in the middle of the season, effectively putting the show out of business until a replacement could be found. A far better answer was a variety bill that could be expanded or contracted at will, depending upon the number of performers available and the specialties they possessed. Using the variety format, something approximating a complete medicine show, including one of the traditional afterpieces, could be performed by three or, if necessary, by two resourceful entertainers.

Medicine show performers belonged to a unique caste with its own rules and traditions and its own place in the hierarchy of traveling entertainment. Their position was not especially exalted. "Stock company actors," said a Toby and Suzy show operator, "felt superior to tent repertoire; musical tab and repertoire actors looked down on each other and both felt superior to carnival people, who felt superior to medicine show people."[4] In part, the status of medicine show performers was low because, unlike entertainers in other outdoor shows, they were expected not only to act and sing but to perform manual labor. Most set up and struck their own stage or tent, hawked candy or medicine during the show, and washed bottles or pasted on labels during their spare time.[5] But they were not necessarily down-at-the-heels vaudevillians, burlesque comedians, or minstrel show performers. Medicine shows often paid as well or better than other outdoor forms, and many entertainers remained by choice in medicine shows for most of their careers,

TO-NIGHT

SPECIAL ATTRACTION IN ADDITION TO REGULAR PROGRAM

MADAM JEWELL

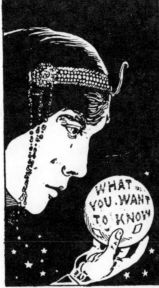

The

Mistress

of

Mystery

The

Wonder

Woman

Presenting a Baffling Demonstration of
MIND READING AND CRYSTAL GAZING

Madam Jewell presents a most awe-inspiring performance. A study of Human Nature and Psychology. SHE WILL ANSWER YOUR QUESTIONS WITHOUT SEEING THEM.

——NO MATTER WHAT YOU WANT TO KNOW——ASK HER——
————————SHE KNOWS————————

A FEW OF THE MANY QUESTIONS YOU MAY WISH TO ASK

Is it advisable to have an operation?   Who stole my automobile?
How often will I marry?   Will I win my law suit?
Have I any enemies?   Will I travel?
When and where will I marry?   Will I sell my stocks?
Will I be wealthy?   When will I get my divorce?

You can depend on getting an answer to any question whether it concerns business, investments, law suits, domestic or social affairs, divorces, estrangements, broken engagements or any other matter.

————ASK HER!!————

Use the form below to write your questions on.   Bring it to the Theatre.

Name ....

Question ....

....

....

Write your question at home.   SIGN YOUR FULL NAME

SEE THIS WONDERFUL WOMAN AT

Special dodger, Lithgow's Vaudeville Concert Company.

gradually learning the traditional "acts and bits" that were part of a standard performance.[6] Some drifted back and forth between medicine shows and tent repertoire, carnivals, or other kinds of traveling shows. Others played medicine shows at the beginning of their careers before moving permanently into vaudeville, legitimate theatre or motion pictures.[7]

A standard middle-sized medicine show company of the teens and early twenties might consist of a lecturer-manager, a sketch team, both of whom also worked singly, a song and dance man, a pianist, and a blackface comedian. Others added a contortionist, a trapeze performer, a magician or a juggler.[8] In 1920 Dr. Heber Becker advertised for a typical vaudeville company, to include "Blackface Singing, Dancing Comedians; must play banjo and guitar. Lady Performer; must sing and dance. Lady to handle and take care of snakes. One good Sketch Team. All people must work in acts and sign contract for season's work."[9] Medicine show entertainers were required to be astonishingly versatile. Shows depended heavily on repeat business during their stay in a community, and in order to get it they were often forced to change their bills every night for a week or two weeks running.[10] At least one company produced a substantially new show every night for forty nights in a row.[11] Advertisements in the trade papers usually specified that performers must be able to "change for a week" or "change strong for ten nights." Since medicine show performers usually appeared two or three times a night, and sometimes more, the size of a performer's repertoire had to be enormous. Bobby Snyder, a late performer, did chalk talks, ventriloquism, rube comedy, blackface comedy, Toby acts, and magic. He also played the guitar and five-string banjo, and performed in all the afterpieces.[12] Frank Golden performed a dozen different specialties and claimed to know by heart a hundred different blackface acts.[13]

Medicine show songs and sketches reflected the sort of casual stereotyping that has always been a commonplace of popular art and entertainment in America. Essentially guileless but often brutal caricatures appeared almost as a matter of course on advertising posters and trade cards, in popular prints, joke books, and patent medicine almanacs, in early films, and in ev-

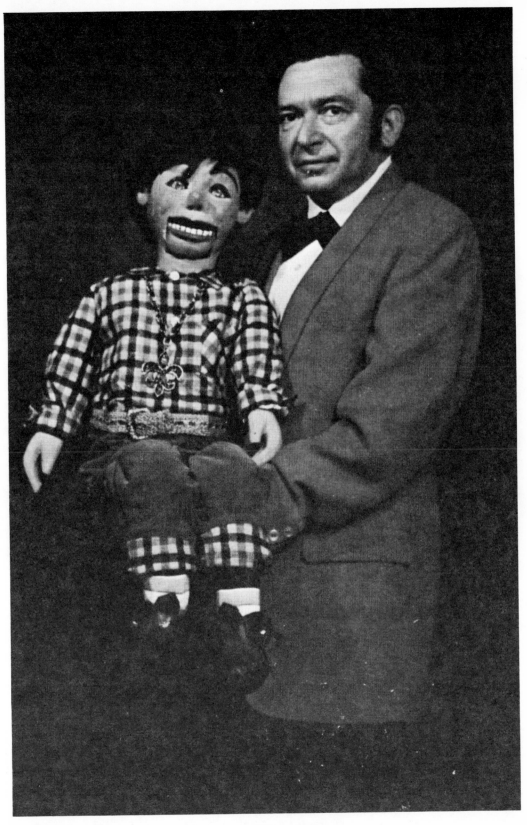

A late medicine show performer, Bobby Snyder.

ery form of variety, burlesque, and legitimate theatre.[14] Women were pilloried, as the old maid, the termagant mother-in-law, and the militant suffragette, along with the effete foreign dude, the absent-minded professor, and the quaint, bib-overalled countryman. Much of popular art was also deeply involved with racial and ethnic stereotypes, and in the medicine show as elsewhere, the Irishman, the Jew, the German, the Italian, and the Negro were transformed into stock comic masks.

It was the blackface comic that dominated most medicine show performances.[15] The blackface comedian, generally called Sambo or Jake, was borrowed from the minstrel show. Like the Interlocutor of the minstrel performances, Jake served as a kind of chief comedian and master of ceremonies, acting in sketches, introducing specialty numbers, playing the banjo and cracking jokes with the straightman. Typically, Jake was dressed in an outfit not too different from the comic tramp costumes of burlesque—huge "slap shoes," gigantic trousers held up by "extra elastic" suspenders that made the comic's pants wobble and bounce at every step, and a shirt or jacket in some violent color combination and outlandish pattern. The blackface makeup—worn on some shows even by Negro performers—was ordinarily the standard theatrical supply house product, although when it was not available an acceptable substitute could be made by burning the cork from the inside of bottle caps and mixing the result with wet ashes. Apache Jack, a medicine lecturer who doubled as his own blackface comic, made up on stage as part of his act, blacking his hands and all of his face except for white circles around his eyes and mouth in under two minutes and gradually shifting from his "Doc" voice to the typical minstrel Jake dialect.[16]

In most troupes Jake also served as "producer" of the show. Traditionally, he bore the responsibility for seeing that performers were "up in all the acts and bits" used by medicine shows and for arranging acts, bits, specialties, musical numbers, and the like into some kind of coherent evening's bill.[17] The medicine show, like the *commedia dell' arte* before it, worked largely out of an oral tradition.[18] Material was casually borrowed from minstrel shows, vaudeville, burlesque, and

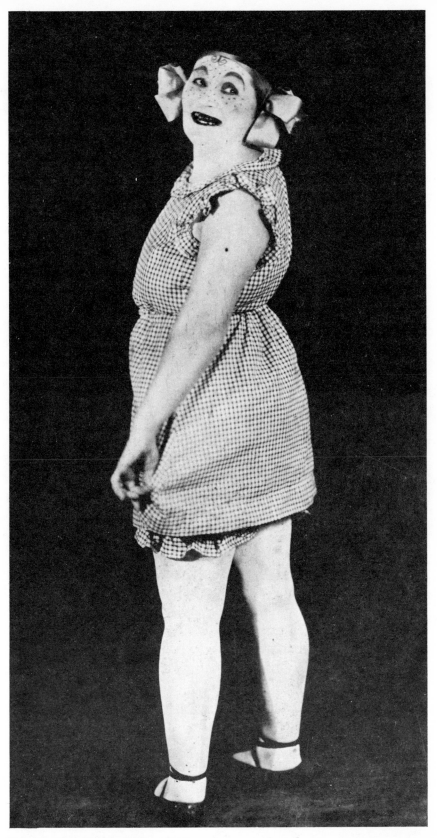

Bertha Wood in a "Silly Kid" costume and makeup, ca. 1929.
ANNA MAE NOELL COLLECTION.

the legitimate theatre, and little of it was written down. It was the function of the blackface comedian as "producer" to know all of the traditional medicine show material, to reconcile one performer's version of a sketch with that of another, and to constantly cut, shape, and organize the bills out of his prodigious memory for acts and bits. Jake, said a former medicine showman, "would say, 'Tonight we're going to open with "The Black Statue" and close with "Three O'Clock Train,"' and everybody on the show knew what was going on. Those people who were in between would do their various specialties, and if a town looked especially good they would add extra material to dress up the show."[19]

A typical medicine show might last two hours and was made up of eight or ten selections, including two or three lectures and their accompanying pitches. A show could start with one of the traditional blackface acts. Most, however, began with a banjo solo or two designed to settle the audience down or a song and dance number featuring the whole cast. Often the second item on the bill was a comedy routine, a rapidfire exchange of jokes and stock bits between the blackface comedian and the straightman. Next came more music or a specialty number—mind reading, magic, or perhaps a sword swallower or ventriloquist—followed by the first pitch and sale of the evening. Soap was often the first item pitched since it was relatively inexpensive and could be used to put a tight-fisted audience in the mood to buy the more expensive tonics and laxatives that appeared later.[20] Next came another act or two, usually a comic bit and a musical act or specialty number, and the second lecture and sale. Finally, after the second lecture, came another bit or specialty number, the prize candy sale, and the traditional medicine show afterpiece, almost invariably a blackface "nigger act" featuring Jake, the straightman, and a ghost.[21]

Because so many medicine show performers had experience with small-time vaudeville or burlesque, or with minstrel companies, side shows or dime museums, a typical bill contained a curious collection of specialty numbers drawn from every kind of popular entertainment. The favorites with small and medium-sized shows were magic acts, songs and dancing, con-

Big pants
Big shoes.
Outlandish colors

"Jake"

"Slap shoes"

Sketch of a typical medicine show Jake character by Anna Mae Noell. COLLECTION OF THE AUTHOR.

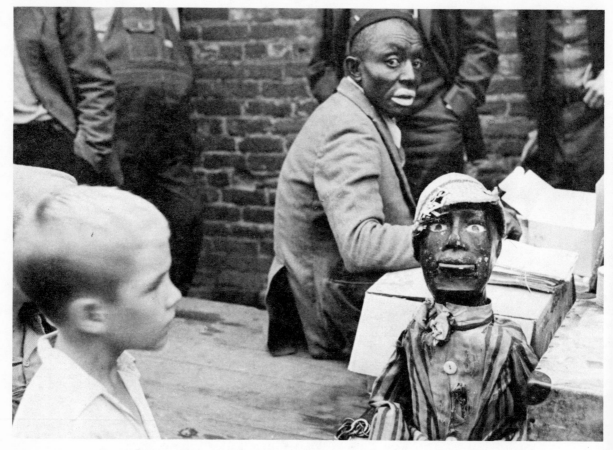

A medicine show Jake and a ventriloquist's dummy used in the
show, Huntingdon, Tennessee, 1935.   LIBRARY OF CONGRESS.

tortionists, ventriloquists, piano and marimba acts, chalk talks,
and fire-eating; but virtually anything that would hold a
crowd appeared on medicine show platforms.[22] Many troupes
used strong men, jugglers, and tumblers; and some large shows
that could carry the equipment employed aerialists and wire
walkers. One of the most famous medicine show specialists was
Frank Lexington, a professional leaper. Onstage at the beginning of his act was an ordinary kitchen table a little larger than
a bridge table. After a very short run from the side of the stage
Lexington would leap over the table without apparent effort.
Then, placing a chair on either side of it, he would leap over all
three objects. Lexington would continue to leap and to add
more chairs until there were three lined up on either side of the

table. Next he placed another chair on top and leaped again, and finally he seated another performer in the chair and vaulted over a total of seven chairs, a table, and the company's blackface comedian.[23]

From the Wild West shows came trick shooting. Claude Gamble, an Illinois journalist, recorded the performance of an entertainer named Diamond Dick, aided by Sambo, his blackface zany. Sambo stood in front of a specially constructed wall of oak planking with an ordinary kitchen match held between his teeth. Diamond Dick made his way to the opposite side of the platform and leveled a rifle at Sambo's head, cooly urging the spectators to be patient in case he should happen to make a mistake the first time. Then he fired and, to tremendous applause from the audience, the match burst into flame. Diamond Dick followed this with other characteristic tricks: firing at a target while sighting in a mirror, and shooting at a swinging target while lying on his back on the stage floor. As the climax of his act, Dick, still prone on the stage floor, shot a playing card from between the lips of the blackface comedian.[24] Other entertainers combined trick shooting with "gun throwing," essentially juggling done with a rifle, or knife throwing, often substituting a mock-terrified Sambo for the pretty girl used as the target in sideshow performances.[25] Probably the most common gun trick—shooting with a rifle or a revolver at glass balls tossed in the air by an assistant—was performed by anyone on the show not otherwise occupied at the moment. The trick was spectacular but amazingly simple since the six-shooter or rifle was carefully loaded with cartridges that contained bird shot instead of a conventional lead slug.[26]

Mind-reading and magic acts were largely borrowed from the variety stage. The range was extremely broad. Harry Houdini presented a relatively elaborate act for Dr. Hill's California Concert Company, a Midwestern medicine show, in 1897, and audiences at the T. P. Kelley shows were treated to a spectacular magic act that included a rainstorm illusion, performed by "Demona, Daughter of the Lightning."[27] At the other end of the scale were the simple acts, often made up of no more than three or four tricks, which any veteran performer was able to present on the spur of the moment. Violet McNeal, for example, hired an out-of-work vaudeville magician to teach her a few tricks to be used along with her medicine pitch. From the professional magician, McNeal learned how to make a silver dollar walk off a man's hand and how to make a playing card, selected by a volunteer from the audience, leave the deck and approach her. Both tricks depended on a hair, attached to a button on the waist of her dress, the free end daubed with shoemaker's wax. The wax was surreptitiously stuck to the card or coin which, as McNeal drew in her abdomen and backed up slightly, moved slowly and mysteriously toward her.[28]

McNeal's third trick, a mind-reading illusion, was if anything less complicated than the other two. The audience was offered a stack of ordinary envelopes. A spectator examined them, chose one, and sealed in it a slip of paper on which he had written a question. The envelope was given to McNeal who placed it in the drawer of a small "spirit" cabinet. As she slid the envelope into the drawer, she swiftly rubbed its face with a sponge dipped in alcohol. The alcohol made the envelope transparent for a few seconds so that the message could be easily read before the drawer was closed for a moment, ostensibly to allow the spirits to do their work. After a suitable amount of hocus-pocus, the drawer was opened and McNeal held the letter against her forehead, stalling to let the alcohol fumes disperse. Then the still-sealed envelope was handed back to the volunteer, the question answered, and the audience considerably impressed by McNeal's apparent extrasensory talents.[29] There were many other variations. Before carbon paper became well known, for example, it was often an essential ingredient of many mind-reading acts. In such acts Sambo generally passed through the audience with an ordinary pad of paper into which small sheets of carbon paper had been inserted at regular intervals. Spectators were asked to write their names and a question on the magical tablet, and the sheet bearing each volunteer's question and his signature was immediately torn off the pad and returned to him. When enough questions had been gathered, the pad was returned to the performer, who launched into a few moments of double talk about the cosmic vibrations of the pad as he surreptitiously

TO - NIGHT!

GERMAN MEDICINE CO.

BIG DOUBLE BILL
   NOTHING LIKE IT EVER SEEN

DONT MISS IT

AMATEUR
CONTEST
TO-NIGHT

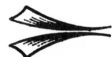

A Silver Cup Given To The Winner.

TO=NIGHT.

Stock dodger, German Medicine Company.

read the carbon copies and then proceeded to answer each question.[30]

Contests and "giveaways" were cheap to operate, they worked well in place of acts and specialty numbers when the company was running low on fresh material, and they had the virtue of directly involving local people in the show—always a sure way to increase attendance. The youngest married couple attending the Jack Roach show was usually presented with a nursing bottle filled with milk and a five-dollar bill, and the oldest couple received a huge basket of groceries tied with a red ribbon.[31] After the first sale of the evening, another show presented purchasers of specially marked medicine bottles with a massive gold watch chain of doubtful pedigree.[32] The so-called "most popular" or "most beautiful" competitions were essentially giveaways of hoary antiquity, dating back as far as the "most beautiful baby" contests used by P. T. Barnum to draw attention to his museum.[33] They were handled in several ways. Generally a competition ran for the duration of the company's stay in a town: on some shows every audience member was entitled to a vote each night; on others purchase of a bottle of medicine or a package of prize candy entitled the buyer to deposit a part of the carton in the ballot box with his nomination for the most beautiful baby or the most popular lady in town.[34] The intent was always the same—to build audiences and to keep excitement running high in the town until the "blow-off," the final night of the show, when the results of the contest were finally revealed and the winner was called to the stage to receive her silver-plated tea set or Indian blanket to the enthusiastic applause of friends and neighbors.[35]

T. P. Kelley ran amateur nights like those staged by many small vaudeville houses, devoting part of the program to quartettes of hymn singers, amateur animal acts, and the perennial recitations and bird call imitations.[36] Many companies with less faith in home talent staged simple contests which depended for their success on placing a group of locals in some sort of ludicrous situation. The German Medicine Company provided showmen with stock dodgers that advertised women's nail-driving and wood-sawing contests.[37] A pie-eating contest was usually done with a dozen small boys from the audience. In one version the boys' hands were tied behind their backs as they attacked pies, smeared with molasses, which dangled from the ceiling by strings, biting away pieces until the first boy to demolish an entire pie was declared the winner.[38] In another version the boys were informed that the pies had been eaten by mistake and that it would be necessary to improvise. Each was provided with a fistful of soda crackers, and the winner was the boy who could still whistle a recognizable tune after consuming his portion of crackers.[39]

Comic songs, bits, and acts were the real heart of the performance. For the most part, medicine show comedy made few claims to undue subtlety or refinement; like the humor in small-time vaudeville and the minstrel show, it tended to be frankly acrobatic and uncomplex. A song popular with medicine shows, for example, was "The Little Red Caboose Behind the Train," which was characteristically performed by Sambo who, during the chorus, turned a lighted cigar backwards in his mouth and blew out streamers of smoke while whistling an imitation of a freight train rounding a curve.[40] Al Lacy's "Billy Goat" song focused on the eating habits, odor, and generally bad behavior of the goat:

One day there was a lady walking through a vacant lot,
She had on her Sunday, go-to-meeting clothes.
But she didn't see the Billy goat, grazing on the spot,
As she stopped to pluck a little rose.
Now Billy saw the lady and he quickly lowered his head.
The lady, she went flying through the air.
Through the hustle and the tustle, you could hear her bustle rustle,
And I should surely know for I was there.[41]

Interspersed with the songs were jokes and quips of ancient vintage. Jingles of the "shave-and-a-haircut-six-bits" variety were traditional on many shows along with fantastic malapropisms, borrowed from minstrel show "stump speeches" and put in the mouth of the blackface comedian. Audiences were treated to such jingles as: "A fly flew in a grocery store,/ He flew in the transom over the door;/ He walked on the sugar and he walked on the ham,/ He wiped his feet on the grocery man."[42] The old adage, "Don't count your chickens before they're hatched," became in Jake's pompous dialect, "You should never speculate upon your juvenile poultry until the proper process of incubation has thoroughly materialized."[43]

The typical medicine show "bit" was a short, single-joke scene, usually performed by the blackface comedian and the straightman, and existing in dozens of variations on medicine shows and in minstrel companies, vaudeville, and burlesque.[44] The "Numbers" bit is characteristic of the kind of short routine done on many shows. The properties were simple—a handful of stage money, and an easel or a chair holding a blackboard on which was written two lines of numbers. On the top line were the numbers from one to five; below it were inscribed the numbers six to nine, and a zero. In a version performed by Anna Mae Noell, the "Numbers" bit went as follows:

STRAIGHT: I got to raise some money to get home on. I came out here to get a job and it didn't pan out so now I'm broke. I fixed this board—maybe I can win a few bets and get some money. (*Enter two comics, Jake and Stooge. Business of nonsense conversation, interrupted by the Straight.*) Say, fellows, how would you like to make a little bet?

JAKE: What kinda bet?

STRAIGHT: I'll turn my back, you pick out a number, then I'll tell you what number you picked.

JAKE: Betcha can't!

STRAIGHT: OK, put your money where your mouth is! How much?

JAKE: Ten!

STOOGE: Ten!

STRAIGHT: Ten!

JAKE: OK, now! Turn yer back! (*Straight turns his back to the board. Jake fumbles around. Finally picks it. Aside, to Stooge:*) There! I bet she don't guess it. I picked the three!

STOOGE: Shhh!

JAKE (*To Straight*): OK, lady (or Mister), I got it.

STRAIGHT: Hmmmm—now, let's see. Was it on the top line?

JAKE: Yep!

STRAIGHT: Was it an odd number or an even number?

JAKE (*Counts. Aside*): One, Two, *Three*. . . . It was an odd number!

STRAIGHT: Ah—ur—was it between Two and Four?

JAKE (*Counts on fingers. Aside*): . . . Two, *Three*, Four. Yep!

STRAIGHT (*Scoops up money.*): The number was Three!

(*Comics talk it over—"How'd she do dat?" etc. Stooge decides Straight can't pick HIS number. Same general business with a new number and the Straight gets the money again. Then the two comics decide the board is such a money-maker they haggle and then buy it. Straight happily counts money and starts to walk away.*)

COMICS (*To Straight*): Hey! Wait a minute! We played the game with YOU—now it's YOUR turn to play with US!

STRAIGHT: I don't want to take your money, boys.

COMICS: That's all right, *etc., etc.* (*Finally, Straight accepts the bet. Comics talk it over.*)

JAKE (*Aside, to Stooge*): If she picks Number One, you tap me one time on the shoulder. If she picks Two, tap me twice. If she picks Nine-hundred-ninety-nine, you beat de devil outa me! (*They bet and the first two times the Comics win. The Straight catches on to their trick but pretends ignorance. Finally, in excited enthusiasm, all three bet all they have on the next guess. The Straight points to the Zero. A lot of funny business follows with Stooge mugging and nearly crying.*)

STOOGE (*To Jake's back, in exasperation*): You ain't no mind reader. You ain't nuthin! Here I done laid ALL my money on you and you cain't tell me what number de lady picked. You know what I ort to do? I know what I'm GONNA do! (*He kicks Jake in the seat.*)

JAKE (*Grabs his seat*): Oh!!!

STOOGE (*Dances happily.*): "O"—dat's de number! "O"! (*Grabs the money. To Jake:*) Boy, if you'd a said "ouch" I'd a killed *you!*

The "Numbers" bit, like most medicine show bits, reads badly. But, of course, "Numbers" was never intended to be read; it is not a play script and cannot be judged as one. "Numbers," like a *commedia dell' arte* scenario, is essentially an outline for action rather than a fully worked-out account of what is to take place on stage. Such phrases as "comics talk it over," "same general business," and "funny business follows" are found whenever bits are written down, and suggest the extent to which they depended on improvisations and interpolations for their vitality. Scraps of dialogue and business floated easily and naturally from one bit to another so that a piece of business used by one comic in "Handy Andy" might appear almost intact as a part of "Simmy Dempsy" or "Little Willie Green." Or the premise of a traditional bit might be altered enough to allow the introduction of a new character or new properties. One company, for example, alternately played two versions of "Little Willie Green" called "Down on the Hats" or "Down on the Chairs," depending on whether or not cheap straw hats were available for demolition at the climax of the sketch. If they could not be found, the bit was reworked so that Jake fell out of a chair each time the bit ordinarily called for a hat to be destroyed.[45]

Some bits, like Bob Noell's version of "The Photograph Gallery" (Appendix A), move in the direction of full-scale acts; and in fact the line between the two types is often not clearly drawn. Often, however, the acts were longer and more complicated, sometimes involved half a dozen characters, depended less clearly on a single joke, and contained some semblance of plot. There were dozens of them: "Brown and Brown," "Widow Bedot," "Black Statue," "Crazy House, or Room 44," "Doctor Shop," "Sir Edwin Booth," and even one named for the king of pitchmen, "Big Foot Wallace."[46] The perennial favorites, known to every medicine show performer and virtually every small-town boy of the early twentieth century, were "Three O'Clock Train," "Pete in the Well," and "Over the River, Charlie" (Appendixes B, C, and D). Like much folk and popular material, their origins are obscure. All three are "nigger acts," trading on the physical dexterity and the malapropisms and mispronunciations of Jake, the blackface comic. Probably all three had their origins in the afterpieces that closed the nineteenth-century minstrel show. In medicine

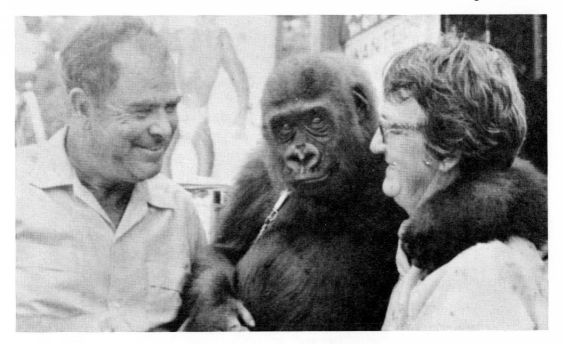

Bob and Anna Mae Noell, late medicine show performers.

COLLECTION OF THE AUTHOR.

show parlance, in fact, "act" and "afterpiece" were used inter-
changeably. Thus, in defiance of all apparent logic, a so-called
afterpiece might open a medicine show or be inserted part way
through the bill. More frequently, however, bits were played
throughout and the afterpiece was reserved for the place of
honor at the end of the show. For most spectators the afterpiece was the best part of the performance, and the announce-
ment that one of the three traditional acts was to be performed
was almost guaranteed to hold an audience through all the
lectures and sales to the very end of the medicine show.

Like the bits, afterpieces were played in countless versions,
and "rehearsal" ordinarily consisted of Jake comparing versions with the straightman and others involved in the act.
There was no need for the performers to know one another.
They merely had to establish the major business that each
used in a particular act and to agree about what was to be kept
and what discarded in their performance together. A rehearsal
might take half an hour or more for a complicated afterpiece
with a large number of characters, or it might be no more

than a few moments of hurried questions and answers between the comic and the straightman: "How do you open the 'Three O'Clock Train'?" "With the Straight explaining." "OK, that's fine with me. Do you do the echo bit?" "Oh, yes! Of course!" "OK, all set."[47]

"Three O'Clock Train" was perhaps the most famous of the afterpieces, an ancient act which also appeared in burlesque and vaudeville and, according to one showman, was to be seen as the "Three O'Clock Coach" as early as the first quarter of the nineteenth century.[48] There were variations without number. The setting, when it existed at all, was a tumble-down and somewhat sinister shanty containing little more than a bench or a pair of chairs facing out across the footlights. In a vaudeville version collected by Douglas Gilbert, the straightman enters, dressed as an eccentric comic with an umbrella, a long coat, and a ridiculously small hat topping a fright wig. The straightman seats himself and begins to scan some letters:

STRAIGHTMAN: If I didn't have this hang-out here I don't know what I'd do. I get the place rent free because the landlord thinks it is haunted. (*Inevitable knock.*) Come in. (*Enter comic.*)[49]

A medicine show version performed by Bert and Bertie Russell starts with the appearance of a third character, who begins the act with considerably more complex exposition:

MAN: My brother wants to sell the old home place and divide the money. I want to keep it and pay him his part. Because we never got along as kids, he's determined to sell to spite me. (*Takes a suitcase, opens it, takes out Ghost robe and puts it on as he continues.*) I've made a bet with him he can't stay all night in this place. I've convinced everyone in the neighborhood the place is haunted so he can't sell it. I intend to show him he can't stay here tonight. (*Exits.*)

STRAIGHTMAN (*Entering*): Well, I never did believe in ghosts, but the old home place sure looks spooky tonight. I've made an agreement with my brother to stay here tonight. If I'm still here in the morning, we will sell the place and divide the money. If I *fail* to stay, he is to pay me what my half is worth and he can keep the place. (*Pauses to look around. Shivers.*) Brrr! It sure is spooky here in the dark alone. Glad the railroad station is close down the road. (*Enter Jake.*)[50]

In Gilbert's script, after the comic enters there follows a gratuitous crossfire about a train, from which the act derives its title:

COMIC (*exaggerated Negro dialect*): Good mawnin'. I just stopped in for some information.
STRAIGHT: I'll try to accommodate you. What is it?
COMIC: What time does the three o'clock train go out?
STRAIGHT: The three o'clock train? Why it goes out exactly sixty minutes past two o'clock.
COMIC: That's funny. The man at the station told me it went out exactly sixty minutes before four o'clock.
STRAIGHT: Well, you won't miss your train, anyway.
COMIC: No, well, I'm much obliged. (*Exits.*)

As Anna Mae Noell performed the same sequence it became a more interesting nonsense dialogue:

JAKE: What time do the three o'clock train leave?
STRAIGHT: At sixty minutes past two.
JAKE: Thought it went past de depot.
STRAIGHT: It runs *on time*.
JAKE: Thought it ran on de track.
STRAIGHT: It goes at three o'clock and is already gone.
JAKE: Train's gone?
STRAIGHT: Yes.
JAKE: Huh. (*Resigned:*) Train's gone!
STRAIGHT: Yes, Jake, the train is *gone*.
JAKE: Er . . . uh . . . are you *sure* the train's gone?
STRAIGHT (*Exasperated*): Yes, Jake, the train is gone. By the way, where you goin'?

JAKE: To Morrow.

STRAIGHT: Oh, that's different, you *can* go tomorrow.

JAKE: I wanna go to Morrow, but I wanna go today.

STRAIGHT: Oh! You want to go to Morrow, Ohio! Well, Jake, that's too bad, because you cannot go to Morrow if you want to go today, for the train that goes to Morrow is already on its way.

The sketch continues in a curious marriage of the comic and the bizarre. The straightman sings a lugubrious song about "the old jawbone on the alms house wall," blue lights flicker and chains rattle offstage, the ghost enters—in one version wearing a derby hat—and Jake and the straightman exeunt, pursued by a ghost.

Scene from *The Medicine Man*, with Jack Benny, Tiffany Productions, 1930. PICTURE COLLECTION, NEW YORK PUBLIC LIBRARY.

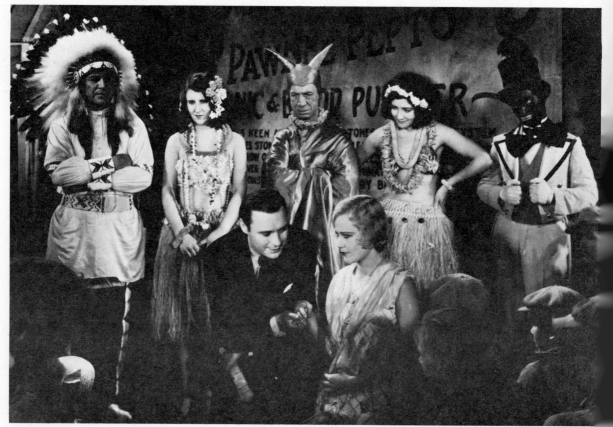

In many respects, the two other great favorite medicine show acts, "Over the River, Charlie," and "Pete in the Well," resemble "Three O'Clock Train." All three are innocently chaotic and filled with the kind of violent clowning that no longer interests most audiences. And all trade on unfeeling stereotypes that are very difficult to swallow today. But in their own time and place they must have had a special kind of power over audiences. It is almost certainly no coincidence that so many medicine shows ended their performances with farces in which white-sheeted apparitions drifted about, bodies were dropped down wells, and ludicrous autopsies with butcher knives and hand saws were commenced on stage. Psychiatrists say that we laugh hardest at the things that frighten us; if this is so, the three famous afterpieces were nothing less than comic reminders to simple people of their own mortality—the doctor's final harangue to the crowd.

10

FOR A BETTER TOMORROW

"Girl came in and told me (very seriously):
'Have you heard about the ninety-five-year-old
lady dying at the hospital?'
"I asked, 'Who was she?'
"'She was taking Hadacol, too. Too bad; and
the Hadacol didn't save her. But they *did* save
the baby.'"

"Salesman came in and said, 'Mrs. Farris, you
read about the bear that was drivin' those people
at Sadelia frantic?'
"I said, 'No. I hadn't heard about it. Did they
catch it?'
"He said, 'Yeah, they caught it. It turned out
to be a mouse that had been taking Hadacol.'"

Herbert Halpert, "Hadacol Stories,"
Kentucky Folklore Record

The last of the big shows did not close for good until 1964, but
the decline of the medicine show had already begun more
than half a century before. In 1906, despite bitter opposition
from patent medicine interests, Congress passed the Federal
Food and Drugs Act, the first federal statute designed to control interstate traffic in food, liquor, and drugs. The Food and

Drugs Act made it a misdemeanor to manufacture, sell, or transport adulterated or misbranded drugs.[1] The effect was to force medicine men to label their products more circumspectly and to make them wary of the kind of fantastic advertising claims that had always been part of the medicine show business. Under the new law, for example, a shipment of Kickapoo Cough Cure was impounded and analyzed, and the company was fined for just the sort of bombast that had always been Healy and Bigelow's stock in trade. The Cough Cure was declared misbranded, "first, because although it contained a certain percentage of alcohol, the package or bottle failed to bear a statement on the label to that effect; second, in that while it was labeled a 'cough cure,' it was not a cough cure, and, third, in that while it was claimed to possess properties recognized by the medical profession as necessary to the proper treatment of diseases of the lungs, it did not, in fact, possess such properties."[2]

State and municipal legislation had always been a headache to medicine showmen and their suppliers, but penalties for violations were not generally too severe and it was often possible to make some sort of deal with local officials. Federal regulation was a different matter altogether. Although some companies blithely continued to manufacture and sell as before, the only sane course was to comply—or at least to appear to comply with the new federal law. In 1912 Texas Charlie Bigelow sold out the Kickapoo Indian Medicine Company to a larger firm. The company that bought Kickapoo was careful to avoid flamboyant, old-fashioned claims. They changed the name of Healy and Bigelow's "cough cure" to the more modest Kickapoo Cough Syrup, announced the contents properly in their advertising, and diffidently pointed out that it was "recommended as an effective expectorant for coughs due to colds, also temporary hoarseness and huskiness of voice due to the same cause."[3] Other firms followed suit. The Suter Remedy Company, which supplied showmen and street workers, began labeling its products far more conservatively, pointing out that Dr. Ranell's Indian Herb Tablets were "for" rheumatism, liver, kidney, blood, and skin diseases, as well as diabetes, indigestion, constipation, dyspepsia, and so-called female trouble—

Advertisement for exposés of patent medicine fraud and quackery.

COLLECTION OF THE AUTHOR.

not, however, that the herbs necessarily *cured* any of these complaints.[4] But later legislation made even such relatively unspectacular statements dangerous. The impoundings, the investigations, and the fines were repeated countless times in the next few years, and many suppliers and showmen began to have second thoughts about the patent medicine business.

Prophets of doom began to foretell the end of the medicine show because of government "interference." Each proposed amendment to the 1906 law was greeted in the trade papers with dark mutterings about "madness" and "radicalism" and plots "to destroy the entire proprietary industry at one swoop."[5] Violet McNeal hired a lawyer to keep her informed of new developments, carefully filing his letters as evidence of her intent to remain within the law while she worked out complicated strategies to circumvent each new piece of legislation.[6] But it was a retreating action. The Food, Drug, and Cosmetic Act of 1938 once again strengthened the laws about manufacture, testing and labeling, and considerably increased penalties for violations. Federal agents began to appear in the audiences of the medicine shows still on the road in the forties, making ominous notes about the lecturer's claims for his remedy.

Unlike the quack who maintained an office and prescribed in private, the medicine showman was forced to sell his remedies in front of dozens and sometimes hundreds of potential government witnesses. Ultimately, the only safe way left to promote medicine in public was not to promote it at all. Milton Bartok, the "Health Evangelist" of the Bardex Show, developed the antipitch to a fine art. "At the end of my pitch," Bartok recalled, "I'd always tell them: 'What does it cure? It doesn't cure a thing. Nature does the curing. Any good physician you go to will tell you the same thing. His cures, or so-called cures, or healing, is with the help of Nature. You break your arm; you go to a hospital. The good doctor puts a splint on it; he wraps it; he does everything. But Nature within your body—if your blood is strong enough, your blood and the marrow of your bones—it will heal. That's why you hear of some people who break a leg or a bone or an arm, it heals in so many weeks—another person, much quicker. You cut yourself. You

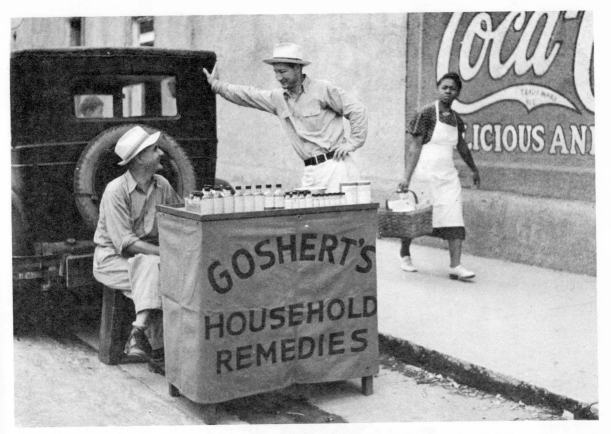

Late low-pitch operator, Port Gibson, Mississippi, 1940.

put mercurochrome, or iodine, or whatever you want to put on it. That doesn't heal it; that prevents infection. Nature heals. There is no medicine that heals anything; it helps Nature. We have wonderful antibodies now—penicillin and so forth. It doesn't heal a thing; it kills the germs. Nature does the curing.'"[7] Most showmen were not as clever as Bartok. The fabulous claims were vital to their pitches and, as the chance for serious trouble increased, they gradually drifted into other, less dangerous forms of outdoor entertainment.

Along with the increasingly rigorous drug legislation came a series of unwelcome economic and social changes. The cost of both drugs and licenses began to climb; the Depression made potential medicine buyers less inclined to spend even small sums freely; and World War II created a crippling shortage of raw drugs, tires, and gasoline. But perhaps most devastating of all was the change that was overtaking medicine show customers. Showmen had always depended on credulous and superstitious audiences. Throughout the new century, the in-

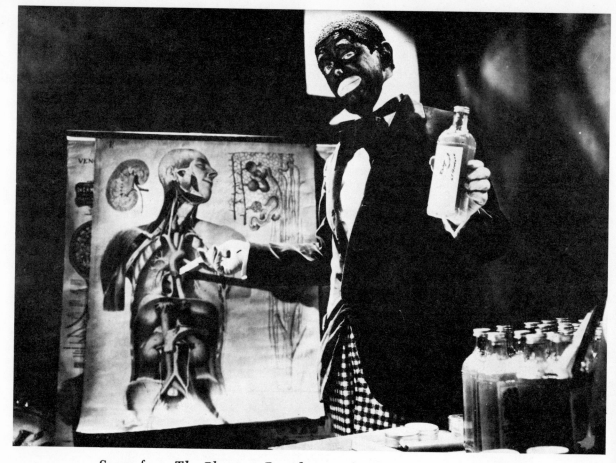

Scene from *The Phantom President*, with George M. Cohan, Claudette Colbert, Jimmy Durante, Paramount, 1932.

creasing sophistication of Americans gradually drove the medicine show into smaller and smaller towns in search of the right sort of customer. Eventually even the smallest towns and villages became unprofitable as country people began to question the patent medicine habit. At the turn of the nineteenth century such mass circulation magazines as *Collier's Weekly* and the *Ladies' Home Journal* had already begun to educate rural readers about patent medicine frauds and quackery through articles by Samuel Hopkins Adams, Edward Bok, Mark Sullivan, Upton Sinclair, and other crusading journalists. The muckrakers were joined by the Anti-Saloon League, the Woman's Christian Temperance Union, and the Temperance League, which denounced the "cheap cocktails" masquerading as patent medicine. Popular magazines and newspapers began to give wide coverage to federal legislation dealing with drug misbranding and abuse. At the same time, the general level of education was rising in rural areas, and the automobile was bringing the previously isolated farmer and his family into contact with the town and its ways, and with modern medicine and pharmacy. By the twenties the archetypal rube—uneducated and gullible—was beginning to disappear, and with him went the medicine show's most valuable customer.

It was not only increasing disillusion about proprietary remedies that spelled the end of the medicine show. Early in the century the Indian show had begun to pall; beginning in the twenties, audiences started to lose interest in the vaudeville performances that had replaced it. For many years the medicine show, along with a few touring companies of *Uncle Tom's Cabin* and an occasional circus, had provided the only more-or-less professional entertainment in many rural areas. Country people were entertainment starved, and they gratefully accepted whatever simple performances came their way. As the automobile increased mobility they began to pick and choose their amusements more carefully. The medicine show inevitably suffered by comparison with the road companies of New York hits which, by the teens, were finding their way to most medium-sized towns and the new motion pictures to be seen in movie palaces at the county seat.

The first American motion picture theatre was opened in McKeesport, Pennsylvania, in 1905. Within four years there were eight thousand more. By 1915 the movies were offering serious competition to vaudeville, burlesque, and the legitimate theatre. In much the same way that they helped to kill vaudeville in the cities, the movies hastened the destruction of the medicine show by providing at a modest price all that a variety show could hope to offer along with the kind of meticulous realism and lavish spectacle that no theatrical company could ever hope to duplicate. To the movies was added radio in 1920, bringing free into the parlors of farmhouses the most skilled and popular singers, musicians, and comedians of the day. In comparison the free show presented by the medicine man and his company began to appear shabby and old-fashioned and perhaps just a little foolish. "Why even the kids

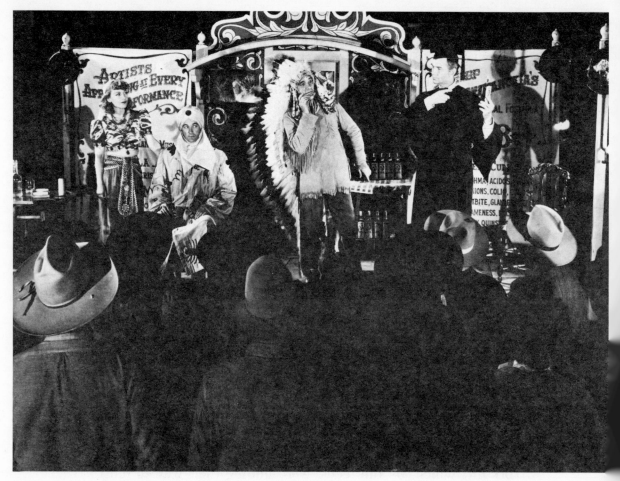

Scene from *Medicine Show*, with William Boyd, Paramount, 1939.
PICTURE COLLECTION, NEW YORK PUBLIC LIBRARY.

have changed," said a showman in the twenties. "In the old days when they came on the lot they were always asking, 'When are the funny men coming out?' Now it's all different; they don't pay much attention to the show on the stage, just keep running around the grounds with a stick or a toy pistol, yelling, 'Bang, bang, bang. I'm William S. Hart, I just shot down the rustlers at the old corral.'"[8]

A number of shows hung on through the thirties, many badly hurt by the advent of talking pictures in 1927 and by the Depression, but still continuing to provide entertainment for the very isolated and the very poor. Some companies were reduced to the role of parasites, appearing in remote areas on the heels of government agents handing out agricultural adjustment checks.[9] By the mid-forties there were perhaps two dozen shows left, half of them sizable and relatively prosperous troupes with a dozen or more employees.[10] The rest were tiny two- or three-man operations.[11] There were many more street-corner pitchmen, but their number was rapidly dwindling, too. By the early fifties there were only eight or ten shows left, most still performing the traditional acts and bits and rather tentatively pitching herb compounds, liniment, and soap.[12]

Most showmen simply retreated in the face of increasing competition from radio and television. A few tried to update the traditional medicine show performance: several companies added country and Western entertainers in an attempt to imitate the immensely successful Grand Old Opry broadcasts; and in the forties Little Doc Roberts of Oklahoma City put his medicine show on the radio to promote Tay-Jo, his patent cure-all.[13] But for the most part owners were not able to combat the inertia that had overtaken the medicine show. There was one extraordinary exception, however, in the person of a Louisiana state senator named Dudley J. LeBlanc, entrepreneur of Hadacol, the most spectacular medicine show remedy since Kickapoo Indian Sagwa. LeBlanc was cut from the same bolt as the great natural geniuses of pitchdom, Healy and Bigelow, Violet McNeal, Big Foot Wallace, and Milton Bartok, and his version of the traditional medicine show was quite unlike anything that had ever taken to the road before in the name of health.

Born of Cajun parents in 1895, LeBlanc operated at one time or another such diverse enterprises as a pants-pressing service, a burial insurance company, and a patent medicine firm that produced two extravagantly euphonious remedies, Happy Day Headache Powders and Dixie Dew Cough Syrup. Happy Day and Dixie Dew were not notable successes. Profits were modest, and in 1941 the Food and Drug Administration began to take an interest in the contents of the headache powder, a batch of which they analyzed, condemned as worthless and probably dangerous, and destroyed. To the irrepressible LeBlanc this was no more than a momentary annoyance, and in 1943 he created his masterpiece, Hadacol, naming it for the Happy Day Company with the addition of the "L" from his

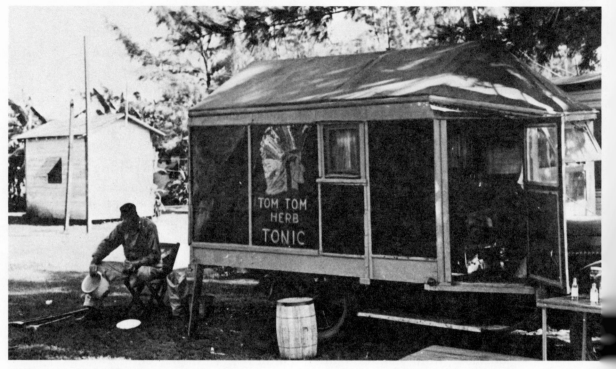

Indian herb tonic pitchman and his house car, Belle Glade, Florida, 1937. LIBRARY OF CONGRESS.

own name. During a bout with arthritis, LeBlanc had been given a series of mysterious but apparently effective injections by his physician. Realizing the potential of the mystery medicine, he filched a bottle from the doctor's office and painstakingly interpreted the label. The injections had been mostly B complex vitamins, and Le Blanc set out to create a vitamin B tonic all his own. The result was Hadacol, an undistinguished remedy which contained, in addition to the B vitamin, honey and 12 percent alcohol.[14] The first batches were stirred up in vats behind LeBlanc's barn by local girls equipped with boat oars. LeBlanc's friends and neighbors sampled the medicine and declared it a success, perhaps because of its appalling taste, which, an associate noted, "some likened to ripe bananas and others to burning rope."[15]

At first Hadacol, like the late Happy Day and Dixie Dew, was aimed at a local market. But shortly LeBlanc began to increase the scale of his advertising. By the end of 1950 he was spending a million dollars a month on a stupendous advertising campaign, which included not only the conventional newspaper and radio advertisements, but such promotional curiosities as glow-in-the-dark T-shirts, Captain Hadacol comic books, and his greatest achievement, the Hadacol Caravan.[16] The origins of the caravan are obscure. As a rural Southern boy growing up in the early years of the twentieth century, LeBlanc must have been well acquainted with the medicine show idea. He could scarcely have escaped exposure to turn-of-the-century shows, and being LeBlanc he almost certainly sought them out as a useful free course in the fine arts of medical double talk and high-pressure salesmanship. Specifically, he seems to have used as his model the Bardex show, run by the most prosperous and imaginative of the late showmen, Milton Bartok. For six weeks, Bartok claims, LeBlanc followed the Bardex shows, carefully storing away ideas about medicine show entertainments and operation that were eventually to be transformed into the Hadacol Caravan Shows.[17]

During the summer of 1950, LeBlanc assembled and sent on the road the first of the gargantuan Hadacol Caravans. Covering 3,800 miles and eighteen Southern states, the caravan entertained on the average 10,000 spectators a night at baseball fields, race tracks, speedways, fair grounds, and football stadiums. On hand was a company like nothing ever seen before in the world of the medicine show. Touring with LeBlanc, who acted as master of ceremonies, were Mickey Rooney, Carmen Miranda, Connie Boswell, Roy Acuff, Minnie Pearl, Chico Marx, and George Burns and Gracie Allen. The Southern tour was followed by a month's stay in Los Angeles, where these show business luminaries were joined by Groucho Marx and Judy Garland.[18] LeBlanc's expenses for the caravan were about $400,000; his profits, according to one account, amounted to more than $3 million.[19] In the following summer he did it all over again on a still more lavish scale, even chartering seventeen railroad cars for his performers, who somewhat cynically dubbed their rolling home The Gravy Train.[20]

Before LeBlanc's Gravy Train finally ran out of steam at the end of the summer of 1951, his passengers were to present the greatest and, for all intents and purposes, the last of the medi-

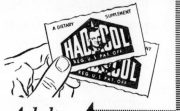

Money CAN'T Buy Admission To This Star - Studded Show!

Admission Is By Box Tops Only!

➤ **1** *for Children* **2** *for Adults* ◄

You'll see these great
featured, headline **stars** in
person . . . on the Hadacol stage:

BOB HOPE*	**MILTON BERLE***
JIMMY DURANTE*	**DICK HAYMES***
CARMEN MIRANDA*	**RUDY VALLEE***
JACK DEMPSEY	**CANDY CANDIDO**
MINNIE PEARL	**HANK WILLIAMS**
JACK BENNY'S "ROCHESTER"*	**SHARKEY**
	And His Kings of Dixieland

*These stars are scheduled in certain cities. Negotiations with additional
top-notch stars are being carried out. See local newspapers for details.

- OVER 14 SCINTILLATING ACTS
- GREAT COMEDIANS
- BIG NAME BANDS
- BRILLIANT VOCALISTS
- PERFORMING CLOWNS
- ACROBATS - JUGGLERS - MAGICIANS
- 50 BEAUTY QUEENS
- DAZZLING FIREWORKS DISPLAY

. . . all preceded (in most cities) by a sensational street parade. It will dazzle and
delight you with its fantastic presentation of Clowns, Calliopes, and twenty
gigantic figures: PREHISTORIC THREE-HEADED WRITHING PYTHON, 100
feet long —— GIANT BALLON LETTERS SPELLING: "H-A-D-A-C-O-L" . . .
with each letter measuring 12 feet high —— BALLOON HUMPTY DUMPTY, 12
feet high —— BALLOON ELEPHANT, 20 feet long —— BALLOON CAT, 11 feet
high —— BALLOON KANGAROO, 14 feet long —— BALLOON SOLDIER, 14
feet high —— BALLOON COW, 20 feet long —— BALLOON INDIAN CHIEF, 14
feet high —— GIANT BALLOON HEAD, 13 feet high —— TEN (10) BALLOON
CLOWN HEADS, each one measuring 4 feet in diameter, etc.

The HADACOL CARAVAN SHOW is intended solely to
entertain our friends, the users of HADACOL. We are anxious to meet you; we are anxious to know you; we wish
we could shake hands with you!
But, because it is not possible to visit with you individually,
and indicate our sincere appreciation for your continued
use of HADACOL—we have organized a great new HADA-

COL CARAVAN SHOW, and invite you, as our customer,
to come and see us. And, we ask that children bring only
one HADACOL box top . . . and that adults bring only two
HADACOL box tops . . . as proof of being a HADACOL
customer.
The HADACOL course is, let's say, 12 bottles. But, we do
not ask that you bring 12 cartons, or 12 box tops to show

that you are a HADACOL customer. No! All we request
is that you merely bring two box tops, if you are an adult,
or, one box top if you are a youngster (under 12 years of
age) when you come to see the HADACOL CARAVAN
SHOW.

NOTE: Cash value of HADACOL Box Top is 1-20 of 1 cent!

Hadacol Caravan Show advertisement.

JAMES HARVEY YOUNG COLLECTION.

cine shows. A typical performance took place at Atlanta's Lakewood Park in August. Long before the caravan arrived in town,
Atlanta was blanketed with newspaper and radio advertising
which promised a fantastic array of events, prizes, and performers. On the afternoon of the show, LeBlanc sponsored
"Storyland Come to Life," a huge parade through the streets
of Atlanta, complete with calliopes, carnival floats, and the
local winner of the Hadacol Beauty Contest.[21] A LeBlanc
parade was a minor Mardi Gras, presided over by the senator
himself in a convertible surrounded by beauty contest winners
from every city along the caravan route who scattered flowers
to the populace. Behind them came more Hadacol beauties on

flower-decked floats and the entire chorus line from the famous Chicago nightclub, Chez Paree. Sharkey and his Kings of Dixieland competed with the calliopes, and above the crowd airplanes towed gigantic banners announcing the big free show to take place that night.[22] Even though advertisements featured such phrases as "Money CAN'T Buy Admission to the Great Star-Studded Show," the caravan performances, strictly speaking, were not free at all.[23] Apparently taking his cue from the breakfast food manufacturers, LeBlanc charged box-tops instead of cash—one Hadacol boxtop for a child and two for each adult. In effect, he had cleverly streamlined the traditional medicine show process by selling his medicine to the audience before they ever set foot in the grandstand.

In a sense, LeBlanc's performances differed little from the sort of thing presented by most late medicine show companies. They were pure escapist entertainment—uncomplex, fast moving, and unabashedly aimed at the taste of the ordinary man—featuring a fairly standard combination of music, dance, comedy, acrobats, and freak acts. Only the traditional blackface afterpiece was missing. But the whole feeling of a Hadacol show was quite different: the scale of the event was far larger; the emphasis was on nationally known stars and personalities; and the acts were conceived with a kind of lavish slickness more typical of the variety shows beginning to fill the screens of seven-inch Du Monts and nine-inch Philcos than of traditional medicine show performances. LeBlanc had created the medicine show spectacular.

Before the Atlanta show began, half a dozen clowns kept the crowd of about eight thousand entertained with acrobatics, stunts, and variations on ancient circus comedy routines.[24] A comic policeman, for example, took a swallow from a giant Hadacol bottle, which caused his eyes to light up behind a pair of prop glasses. Another clown grabbed the bottle, and as he drank, his nose lit up and glowed red. After the clowns, LeBlanc himself appeared on the field, emerging from a huge Cadillac to shake hands with the performers and wave to the crowd that was beginning to fill the Lakewood Park grandstand. As the senator departed, the show officially opened with Tony Martin's band playing a Gershwin medley. Next, Cesar

Romero, the master of ceremonies, told one of the ever-so-slightly-shady Hadacol stories that were sweeping the country and introduced the Dorothy Dorben dancers of Chicago's Chez Paree, who performed with multicolored Hadacol balloons. The dancers were followed by Sharkey Bonano and his dixieland band which played a version of LeBlanc's theme song, a rather thinly veiled musical celebration of the tonic as an aid to sexual prowess, "The Hadacol Boogie."

Bonano's act ended with a song and dance routine by two Negro dancers, Pork Chops and Kidney Stew. They were followed by an acrobatic act, and Larry Logan, a harmonica player, who for culture's sake entertained the audience with Enesco's First Roumanian Rhapsody. To liven up the proceedings again, Emile Parra told a series of Hadacol stories centering around male potency and danced a violent version of the "Darktown Strutters' Ball" complete with back bends and wild gyrations to demonstrate what was possible after taking Hadacol. Next came a comic "Before and After Hadacol" act featuring a midget and Ted Evans, the English giant. Dick Haymes sang several romantic and patriotic songs, and Ann Maucele, a lady tumbler, performed.

In the last half of the show, Carmen Miranda appeared with her Bando da Lua boys, singing a few songs and joking about the bananas in her hat. The Dorben dancers performed again in an Indian number, and Romero introduced the winner and runner-up in the Atlanta section of the Hadacol Beauty Contest, along with the winners of prizes for collecting the most Hadacol boxtops. Next came a juggler, and comedian Candy Candido who sang and cracked a few Hadacol jokes. Then Jack Dempsey appeared in a kind of nonact in which he extolled the virtues of Dudley LeBlanc as patron of the Hadacol caravan, friend of his home state, the South, and the nation, and the next governor of Louisiana. To his campaign pitch for LeBlanc, Dempsey added a sales talk for defense bonds before turning over the platform to the final featured act of the evening, Hank Williams and his hillbilly group with the comedian, Cousin Minnie Pearl. Then most of the company returned to the stage for a farewell song, and the evening ended with a lavish show of fireworks, culminating in a set piece of the American flag side by side with another display that spelled out in letters of fire LeBlanc's favorite motto, "Hadacol for a Better Tomorrow."

But tomorrow was not to come. Shortly after the Atlanta show LeBlanc announced the sale of the company to a New York firm. Almost immediately the new owners denounced the senator for having juggled the Hadacol books by concealing two million dollars in unpaid bills and listing as "accounts receivable" another two million which, in fact, was simply Hadacol out on consignment. Much of it was rapidly returning. In spite of the shows and the other spectacular promotional devices, the Hadacol boom was over once and for all. Americans turned back to their television sets; they had seen all of the Hadacol shows they cared to see and they had bought all the Hadacol they were going to buy. LeBlanc knew it, and like any good pitchman he had doused his torches and driven away just in time.

In the wake of his departure were to be found a number of unhappy medicine showmen. The giant Hadacol Caravan had represented the last bit of impossible competition for most of the handful of shows still operating in the early fifties. Lecturers and performers began to look for new jobs in carnivals, circuses, and amusement parks. Many were getting old. They retired to Gibsonton, Florida, or one of the other sunny towns favored by entertainment people—some with considerable fortunes, many into dreary rooming houses and trailer camps. The Keen-O-Tone show closed in 1951; the Ja-Dex show lasted until the late fifties; Milton Bartok's big Bardex show, which employed more than thirty musicians and performers, closed in 1960.[25] By this time there was little interest among outdoor amusement people in pitching and medicine shows. There were virtually no shows left and almost every city had long since barred pitchmen from working doorways and downtown street corners and parking lots. In 1961 *The Billboard* changed its name and its format and reemerged as *Amusement Business;* with interest at a low ebb it was decided, after more than half a century, to abandon the medicine showmen's column, "Pipes for Pitchmen."[26] Three years later Bartok opened his show again for a single season and then closed down for good.[27] By the middle of the sixties the medicine show had simply ceased to exist.

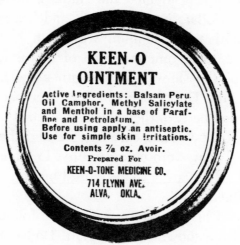

Ointment tin, Keen-O-Tone Medicine Company.

COURTESY OF BILL SMITH.

The end came, in large part, because of competition from other forms of free entertainment. The premise of the medicine show was that a free performance would sell a product. The premise was a sound one and radio and television merely borrowed it and developed it on a scale far beyond anything dreamed of by the traveling medicine showman. Ironically, in doing so they helped to put the medicine show out of business. But something of the old spirit continued. "Nowadays the props have been improved and the jargon refined; but the pitchman's approach has not altered measurably," says Long John Nebel, an ex-pitchman who graduated to radio and television.[28] And of course he is right. Just behind the bland, smiling figure of the television announcer stands the ghost of a turn-of-the-century medicine showman, his silk hat tilted at a

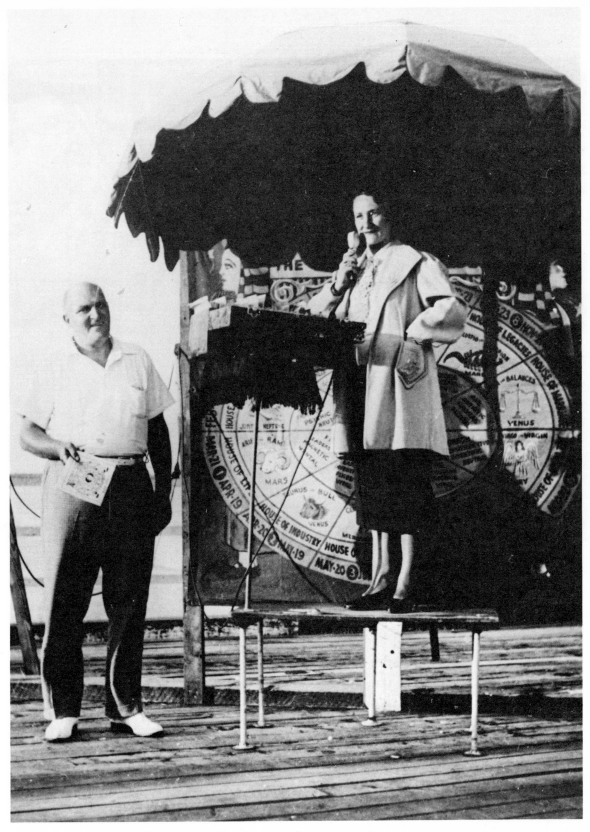

Harry and Elsie Busch, a late pitch team, 1938.

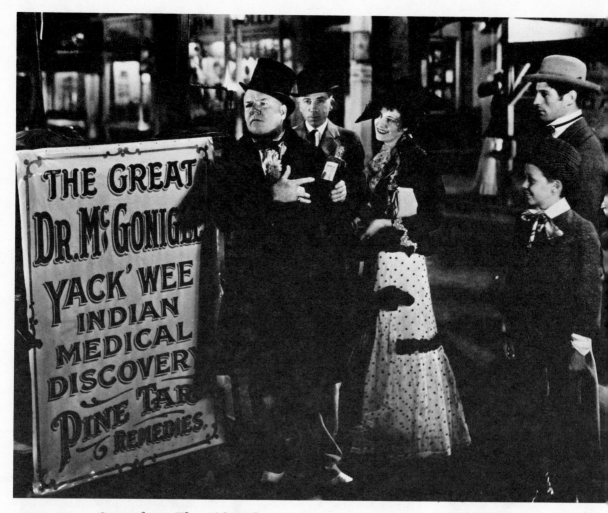

Scene from *The Old-Fashioned Way*, with W. C. Fields and Baby
Le Roy, Paramount, 1934.

rakish angle and his shirt front ablaze with diamonds. "Step
right up," he seems to say, "here you are! You may not have
cinderella but if you haven't it's a cinch you've got something
else and no matter what it is this little box will save your
life. . . ."[29]

APPENDIXES A-D

A Medicine Show Bit and Three Acts

The "Photograph Gallery" bit, "Pete in the Well," and "Over the River, Charlie" were played on medicine shows by Bob and Anna Mae Noell and were transcribed by her for this book. "Three O'Clock Train" was collected by Douglas Gilbert and appeared in his *American Vaudeville*.

APPENDIX E

A Glossary of Pitchmen's Terms

APPENDIX A

The Photograph Gallery
(Bob Noell's Version)

Cast
Straight
Jake

Properties

Bogus camera; black cloth to use with camera; two-sided "photograph" with sketch of Jake on one side and a donkey's head on the other; a table; a chair.

STRAIGHT: I've rigged up a bogus camera and as soon as I can rope someone in, I'll raise enough money to get out of this town. Here comes someone now. (*Stands erect and looks important as Jake enters.*)

JAKE: I brung 'em.

STRAIGHT: You brought *what?*

JAKE: 'Taters.

STRAIGHT: You brought potatoes?

JAKE: Yep. I put 'em in the cellar.

STRAIGHT: I didn't order any potatoes!

JAKE: Yes, you DID!

STRAIGHT: That's a laugh! Whatever made you think I ordered potatoes?

JAKE: I seen it on the sign out there: "POTATOES TAKEN HERE."

STRAIGHT (Laughs): Oh! hahaha, Jake, that doesn't say "potatoes." That sign says "Photographs Taken Here."

JAKE: Oh, I ain't got none of them!

STRAIGHT: No, you don't understand! This is a photograph gallery! Tell you what I'll do! I'll take your picture.

JAKE: No, you don't! You don't get no picture of mine. I done told you I ain't got none!

STRAIGHT: Jake, how much are the potatoes in the cellar?

JAKE: Three dollars! Pay me or I'll leave!

STRAIGHT: Now, Jake. Wouldn't you like to have a nice picture of yourself to give to your girl?

JAKE: Ha ha! Dat would be nice, wouldn't it? But where I gonna get one?

STRAIGHT: Right here. That's what I do. See that black box over there?

JAKE: Yeah, I see it all right. What is it?

STRAIGHT: That's the camera.

(*Jake sidles cautiously around the Straight, putting the Straight between himself and the camera and then peeks at the camera. Business.*)

STRAIGHT: What's the matter Jake?

JAKE: I ain't never monkeyed around with no cannon before.

STRAIGHT: Oh Jake, don't be silly. Now, I can make a picture that will look *just like you!*

JAKE: You can? How much do dey cost?

STRAIGHT: Well, the first dozen is ten dollars; the second dozen is five dollars; and the third dozen is free.

JAKE: I'll take some of the third dozen first.

STRAIGHT: No, Jake. But I'll tell you what I *will* do; I'll make you *one* picture for the potatoes in the cellar!

JAKE: Will it look like me?

STRAIGHT: I promise.

JAKE (*Business*): Haha, gonna give it to my gal!

STRAIGHT: OK, Jake, please sit in front of the camera.

(*Jake starts to exit.*)

STRAIGHT: Wait a minute, Jake, where are you going?

JAKE: I dunno, but I ain't sittin' in front of no *cannon*.

STRAIGHT: JAKE! This is the box that makes the picture, not a *cannon*. It's a camera. Now please take a chair.

JAKE: Don't mind if I do. (*Picks up chair and starts to exit while the Straight has his head under the black cloth.*)

STRAIGHT (*Coming out from under the cloth*): Here! Here! What are you doing?

JAKE: You said take a seat.

STRAIGHT: No I meant "take a chair and sit down."

(*Jake sits on floor with chair in lap, muttering happily, "gonna give it to my gal!" Straight comes out from under cloth several*

times, each time in a bewildered search for his hyperactive
"subject." Finally the Straight finds him.)

STRAIGHT: JAKE! What are you doing on the floor?

JAKE (*Angrily*): You *said* to take a chair and sit down! I'se
    done what you SAID!

STRAIGHT: No! No! No! (*Exasperated:*) I mean, "SIT ON THE
    CHAIR"!

JAKE: Why the devil didn't you say so in the first place! (*To*
    audience:) Gonna give it to my gal, ha ha.

(*Straight is under the black cloth again, "focusing" on Jake.*
Waves hand over camera to Jake. Jake laughs and says, "Dat's
nice, she's waving at me." Gets up, shakes hands with the
Straight. Straight untangles self from cloth and angrily shouts,
"What on earth do you think you're doing?")

JAKE: You was waving yer hand at me.

STRAIGHT (*Trying to contain temper, softens voice menacingly*
    and says): Jake, when I wave my hand this way (*palm*
    down), it means LOWER, LOWER, LOWER. When I wave my
    hand *this* way (*palm up*), it means HIGHER, HIGHER,
    HIGHER. And so forth and so on (*waves hand side to side*).

JAKE: Hope there ain't too much "so forth and so on."

(*Straight, under the cloth again, waves his hand "higher,*
higher, higher." Jake raises himself a little each time the hand
is waved, and finally ends up sitting perched on the chair
back with his feet on the seat, still chuckling, "Gonna give it to
my gal, haha." Straight untangles again.)

STRAIGHT (*Angrily*): Jake, we're never going to get this picture
    made if you don't stop your foolishness. What are you
    doing NOW?

JAKE: You SAID "Higher," and this is the highest I could get.

STRAIGHT: Please, Jake, SIT DOWN.

(*Jake mumbles "gonna give it to my gal" to the audience as he*
sits. The Straight waves his hand "lower, lower, lower." Jake
keeps moving down until he is lying flat on the floor.)

JAKE: Doggone it, quit waving—I cain't *git* no lower!

STRAIGHT (*Untangles. Almost cries*): Jake, I'm going to try
    it one more time. Please—*You* sit still and *I'll* move the
    camera.

(*Jake grins at the audience: "haha, gonna give it to my gal."*
Straight gets under the cloth again. He moves the box up and

down trying to "find" his subject. Meanwhile, Jake jumps up, yelling.)

JAKE: HOT DOG! I found another one!

STRAIGHT (*Untangles*): Another *what?*

JAKE: I found another pin with the point pointing toward me! That's good luck! My Ma says if I find a thousand pins with the point pointing toward me I'll get a brand-new automobile. I done found nine hundred and ninety-eight pins! All I need is two more!

STRAIGHT (*Stares at Jake for a moment and shakes head*): Well, OK. Now are we ready to try again?

JAKE: Oh, yeah. De picture. Yeah—just need *two more pins!* Ain't dat sumpin? (*Straight goes under. More business with camera. Jake jumps up, excited.*) DOGGONE! Dere's another pin with the point right toward me!

(Straight untangles, sneaks behind Jake. Business of taking pin out from under collar and fixing it in chair so Jake will "get the point." All the while Jake is in ecstasy over his luck, mumbling, "All I need is ONE MORE PIN." *Lots of funny business here of Straight watching in anticipation as Jake starts to sit, then gets up. Several tense moments. Each time Jake rises he asks the Straight a new question: "Will it look like me?" "Will my gal like it?" "I ain't gonna pay if it don't look like me!" "You sure she'll like it?" "Can I get it right away or do I hafta wait?" Finally, when he sits, Jake bounces straight up with a yowl.)*

STRAIGHT (*Snickering*): What's the matter, Jake?

JAKE: I found the other pin. (*Pause for laughter.*) With the point right toward me.

STRAIGHT: OK, now let's get back to the picture.

(Jake, rubbing the seat of his pants, turns and runs his hand all over the chair seat, then slides across the seat and says "ahh". Turns to audience, smiles, and says, "Gonna give it to my gal, haha!" Straight goes under the cloth, then moves the camera. Jake peers into it inquisitively. Straight untangles.)

STRAIGHT: Jake, you were looking right into the camera. That's bad. Let's see. Oh, yes—do you see that fly on the wall behind the camera?

JAKE (*Cranes his neck*): No, I don't see him, but I know he's there.

STRAIGHT: If you can't *see* him, *how* do you know he's there?

JAKE: I can hear him walking.

STRAIGHT: Jake! I know you can see that fly. NOW, KEEP YOUR EYE ON THAT FLY.

(*Straight goes under the cloth just as Jake's fly takes flight. Jake stands and moves his head rapidly, watching the fly's erratic flight, then, as the Straight untangles and watches, faces the audience and says, "Cain't be done! Cain't be done!"*)

STRAIGHT: *What* can't be done?

JAKE: Cain't keep my eye on the fly.

STRAIGHT: Why not?

JAKE (*Pointing to a child in the audience*): That little boy down there swallowed it.

STRAIGHT: Jake, enough of this nonsense! See the knothole on the wall?

JAKE: Yep.

STRAIGHT: OK, keep your eye on that knothole. (*Goes under.*)

JAKE: Doggone! Always did like to peep through knotholes— see a lot of funny things that way. (*He walks over to the wall and puts his eye to the knothole. Straight untangles and asks Jake what he is doing. Jake argues.*)

STRAIGHT: Jake, just sit still. (*Goes under. He slaps the table loudly under the camera and pulls out the hand-sketched portrait of Jake.*)

JAKE (*Angrily*): Dat don't look like me!

STRAIGHT: I say it DOES!

JAKE: DON'T!

STRAIGHT: DOES!

JAKE: DON'T! Etc.

(*Finally the Straight appeals to the front row, which was always made up of children.*)

STRAIGHT: Doesn't this look like Jake?

JAKE: No!

CHILDREN: Yes!

JAKE: No!

CHILDREN: Yes!

JAKE (*Finally, to Straight*): All right den, if DAT (*indicating the picture*) looks like ME, den DIS (*flipping the picture to reveal the donkey head on the back*) looks like YOU.

APPENDIX B

Three O'Clock Train
(A Vaudeville Version Collected by Douglas Gilbert)

Cast
Comic [Jake]
Straight

Setting
A bare and dingy room

STRAIGHT: If I didn't have this handout here I don't know what I'd do. I get the place rent free because the landlord thinks it is haunted. (*Inevitable knock.*) Come in. (*Enter comic.*)

COMIC (*Exaggerated Negro dialect*): Good mawnin'. I just stopped in for some information.

STRAIGHT: I'll try to accommodate you. What is it?

COMIC: What time does the three o'clock train go out?

STRAIGHT: The three o'clock train? Why, it goes out exactly sixty minutes past two o'clock.

COMIC: That's funny. The man at the station told me it went out exactly sixty minutes before four o'clock.

STRAIGHT: Well, you won't miss your train anyway.

COMIC: No, well, I'm much obliged. (*Exits.*)

STRAIGHT: Curious sort of chap. (*Picks up banjo and strums quietly as Comic reenters.*)

COMIC: Excuse me, which is the other side of the street?

STRAIGHT: Why, the other side of the street is just across the way.

COMIC: That's funny. I asked the fellow across the street and he said it was over here.

STRAIGHT: Well, you can't depend on everything you hear.

COMIC: No, that's so.

STRAIGHT: Well, you've got plenty of time to make your train. Sit down a while.

COMIC (*Seating himself, and scanning the wretched room*): Nice place you have here. Nice comfortable place.

STRAIGHT: Yes, I get the place for a very reasonable rent. Know why I get it so cheaply?

COMIC: You don't pay the rent.

STRAIGHT: No, no. It's because the place is haunted. (*Comic looks round uneasily.*)

STRAIGHT: But you're not afraid of ghosts?

COMIC: Oh, no. I'm not afraid of ghosts. My grandmother used to keep a ghost boardinghouse. Some of my best friends are ghosts. (*Looks nervously around.*)

STRAIGHT: Well, I'm glad to hear that because this house is full of ghosts.

COMIC: When do the, that is, when, er, where are they, these, er . . . ?

STRAIGHT: Oh, they're liable to come in any time.

COMIC (*Shuddering*): Right in here?

STRAIGHT: Oh, yes, right in here. They just waft in and waft right out again.

COMIC: They, they waft, do they? (*Looks round uneasily.*)

STRAIGHT: What's the matter?

COMIC: I thought something was wafting.

STRAIGHT: Well, you wouldn't care, would you?

COMIC (*With exaggeration*): Oh, no. I wouldn't care.

STRAIGHT: Like to hear a good song?

COMIC: Yes, I always liked music. Something lively.

STRAIGHT: All right, I'll sing you a good lively song.

COMIC: Something to cheer us up?

STRAIGHT: Oh, yes. Something very cheerful. (*Sings, in dismal wail:*)

The old jawbone on the alm's house wall.
It hung fifty years on that whitewashed wall.
It was grimy and gray, and covered with gore,
Like the souls of the sinners who'd passed there before.

Chorus: Oh, the old jawbone, the jawbone, etc.

(*Chains rattle and weird noises are heard backstage as stage lights dim. Comic shivers in terror.*)

STRAIGHT: What's the matter with you?

COMIC: Oh, nothing. Nothing at all. I'm just enjoying the music. That's a nice lively song.

STRAIGHT: Oh, wait till you hear the second verse. (*Sings, still in dismal wail:*)

At twelve o'clock near the hour of one,
A figure appears that will strike you dumb.
He grabs you by the hair of the head,
And he grabs you about until you are dead.

(*Offstage noises and wails. Straightman rises and ghost enters and straightman exits, singing:*)

Oh, the old jawbone . . .

(*Ghost slithers to chair vacated by Straightman and sits beside Comic unknown to him because he has not seen the entrance.*)

COMIC (*Still unaware of ghost*): Why not sing something we both know? We'll sing it together. Yours is a good song but I don't like the way it ends. (*Ghost nudges Comic.*)

COMIC: I wasn't asleep. I was just listening to the music. Is it most time for them ghosts to waft? (*He looks casually to one side and sees part of the white sheet. He follows his glance, takes in ghost completely, and rises, horrified, as ghost rises with him. He pulls the string of fright wig and hair stands straight up. Recovering somewhat, Comic edges away and then dashes round stage, and ghost, his finger pointing at Comic, pursues. As ghost gradually gains on Comic, Comic exits, diving through breakaway window.*)

APPENDIX C

Pete in the Well
(Jack Roach's Version)

Cast
Jake
Straight
Pete

Setting
A pawnshop

STRAIGHT: I'm *most* annoyed tonight! I forgot to lock my safe last night and I have just discovered that someone has stolen twelve cents out of the safe. An old dime and two pennies. Keepsakes. I'll call Jake and Pete and I'll bet I'll get to the bottom of this! Jake! Come up here!

JAKE (*Enters*): Yas'm (or Yassir).

STRAIGHT (*Repeats what happened and asks*): Now, what I want to know is DO YOU KNOW WHAT HAPPENED TO MY OLD COINS?!

(*Jake denies—Straight presses—Jake denies until finally he yields by saying, "If you don't tell him I told you, I'll tell you." —Looks offstage both directions, then sidles up to Straight and in a hoarse whisper says, "Last night I went to the carnival and I saw Pete and his girl friend. They were licking a 1¢ lollipop each and riding on the 5¢ merry-go-round. So there goes your 12¢."*)

STRAIGHT: Aha! I thought so! I'll just call him up here and fire him!

JAKE: Let me outta here first!

STRAIGHT: No! You stay here! (*Turns and calls:*) Pete!

PETE (*Offstage—in a surly, rough voice*): What do you want?

STRAIGHT: Come up here right away—it's very important!

PETE: I'll come when I get good and ready!

STRAIGHT: You'll come NOW!

PETE (*Enters, and again says*): OK, I'm here. What do you want?

STRAIGHT: I understand you were on the merry-go-round with your girl last night. Where did you get the money?

PETE: Who told you I was on the merry-go-round?

STRAIGHT: A little bird told me.

PETE: Oh, yeah? I'll bet it was a damned BLACK Bird! (*Starts running after Jake menacingly. Jake flees all around the Straight, as he yells, "Hold 'im! Hold 'im!" When Straight DOES hold Pete, Jake takes up a sparring stance and says, "Let 'im go! I ain't scared of 'im! Let 'im go!" Straight lets Pete go and Jake turns tail, again yelling, "Hold 'im!" This is done two or three times. Then Straight says, "Enough of this! Pete, you're fired!"*)

PETE (*Aside to audience*): Too damned late, I quit ten minutes ago—(*Exits.*) I'm coming back to rob this joint tonight.

JAKE: Did you hear that? Did you hear what he said?

STRAIGHT: No—what did he say?

JAKE (*In awed amazement—wide-eyed*): He said he's coming back to rob this joint tonight.

STRAIGHT: He DID, did he! *Well*—we'll just see about that. I never did like that guy anyway. Now, Jake, here's what we will do—you hide over there and I'll hide over here. You take the broom and hit him over the head if you have to. I'll take the gun, and we'll just lay for him. (*They hide in opposite wings.*)

(*Enter Pete—stealthily creeping, looking to right and left. Pulls drawer out of table as Jake comes up behind with brush end of broom and swats him just as the Straight fires the gun. Pete falls flat on his back with his arms and legs outstretched.*)

JAKE: Lordy! You done killed him!

STRAIGHT: I didn't kill him, Jake. You did. (*While Jake is protesting his innocence, Straight removes broom and puts gun in Jake's hand.*) I had the broom. YOU shot him!

JAKE: No siree—I had the broom—Yi! How did I get that thing?! (*Gingerly lays gun on table and backs away.*)

STRAIGHT: Jake, we've got to move fast. Now that you've killed him, the Pinkerton detectives will be after you.

JAKE: Oh, Lordy, I don't want no Pink-eyed detectives after me!

STRAIGHT: Well, here's what we must do, then. We will get rid of the body, then take inventory and run away to Canada. That's our only chance!

JAKE: OK. What do you want me to do?

STRAIGHT: Get rid of the body.

JAKE: How I gonna do dat?

STRAIGHT: There's an old well in the backyard. Uncover it— throw him in—throw in a lot of rocks, then cover it back. Hurry! We haven't got a minute to lose. (*Exits.*)

JAKE: Oh, Lordy, I gotta get rid of the body. Look at that son of a gun! Died jest like a pair of scissors—all spread out. OK, here goes. (*He pulls feet together and Pete's arms fly straight up. Jake jumps back in fright. Then he stands astride Pete and pushes his arms back down to his sides. Pete's feet fly up, kicking Jake in the buttocks. Jake jumps away in fright again. Finally he pushes Pete's feet to the floor again, causing Pete to sit up. Jake adjusts Pete so that he is facing the audience. Then he sits down by Pete and apologizes, saying—"I swear, Pete, I didn't shoot you. I'm sorry about the whole mess." As he talks, Pete slowly turns his head and looks at Jake who discovers the staring eyes and pushes the head back around to the front. Repeat. Then Jake goes and sits on the other side. Pete turns that way. Repeat. Finally Jakes says, "OK, I gotta get rid of the body." He puts his arms under Pete's arms, lifts him to a standing position, and bounces him along to the side of the stage where he carefully props him against a wing. In bouncing Pete, Jake loses his hat—it falls just out of reach. He tries to pick it up, but Pete teeters forward, about to fall. Repeat. Finally, Jake lies down on his back, holding up the teetering Pete with his feet. Jake grabs his hat and puts it on. Jake gets up, turns his back to Pete, and reaches over his shoulders to carry him on his back. Pete ducks down. As Jake turns to look at him, Pete stands straight again. Repeat. The third time, Pete escapes off the stage. Jake yells for Straight, "Hey, Boss! Hey, Boss!"*)

STRAIGHT: Well, Jake, I see you got rid of the body.

JAKE (*Bewildered—looking around worriedly*): Yas'm—I got rid of the body, all right.

STRAIGHT: Now, Jake, you sit here at the table and take this tablet and pencil and write down what I call off to you.

JAKE: But I can't see! It's dark in here.

STRAIGHT: Well, then, light a candle. (*Exits. Jake lights the candle, which is already sitting on the table. The table is covered to the floor with a cloth and a fourth person is under the table manipulating the spooky candle. The Straight calls from offstage:*) "Three Chickering Pianos."

(*Jake writes laboriously as he mutters, "Three chickens on a Piano," then watches in fascinated horror as the candle "grows" taller and taller and taller. He yells, "Hey, Boss!" Straight enters.*)

STRAIGHT: What's the matter, Jake?

(*Jake blubbers at the now normal-size candle. Straight fusses a little and exits as Jake sits down again.*)

STRAIGHT (*From offstage*): "Seventeen monkey wrenches."

JAKE: "Seventeen wenches." (*Then Jake watches the candle slide across the table. He calls the Straight. The candle returns to its place. The Straight fusses, then says, "Jake bring the candle over here and let me see what you've written down." Jake brings the candle.*)

STRAIGHT: Hold it so I can see. (*Pause.*) Higher. Higher, Jake. (*Jake now looks like the Statue of Liberty, with his arm fully extended over his head. Straight looks up and says, "Oh, Jake, LOWER!" Jake lowers it below reading level. Straight says, "Lower! Lower!" Looks up and says, "Jake! Hold it betwixt and between!" Jake turns back to audience, bends over and holds candle flame to seat of pants, then jumps and howls in pain. Straight finally gets Jake's hand in the correct position and says:*) "Jake! Who said anything about chickens on a piano?"

JAKE: You did. You was right in dat room over there (*extends arm*) when you said it.

(*Ghost enters, puts head under arm and looks at Jake. Jake pantomimes fear, then slowly looks at ghost—clamps arm down hysterically, dropping candle as he beats himself on the arm. The ghost has escaped.*)

STRAIGHT: What's the matter with you, Jake?

JAKE: I saw him—Pete. Right here!

STRAIGHT: Stop the nonsense. We have no time to lose. Get with it, man! What else did you write? Oh, Jake! I never said anything like this! I said MONKEY wrenches.

(*Ghost crawls in. Jake's legs are spread wide enough for the ghost to lie down on his back looking up at Jake as he snatches and pulls Jake's pants legs repeatedly. Jake has trouble keeping his pants on and holding the candle. He sees the ghost, who escapes. Jake sits down violently where the ghost had been. Straight fusses. Jake gets up. Straight gives Jake the paper and says, "We'll do the rest of it now, but this must be done over." The ghost comes in again and taps Straight on the shoulder, then points offstage. The terrified Straight exits silently. Jake is still arguing—"You was right over there, etc." Ghost in somber tones quavers, "It's all wrong."*)

JAKE: You got a cold or sumpin, Boss? Your voice sure changed sudden-like! (*Jake slowly looks around at the ghost, then runs offstage with the ghost riding on his back.*)

APPENDIX D

Over the River, Charlie
(Anna Mae Noell's Version)

Cast
Dr. Kelly (Doting, protective father)
Kitty Kelly (His beautiful daughter)
Kitty's Suitor, "Charlie"
The Houseboy, "Jake"

Setting
The Living Room of Kelly's Home

DR. KELLY (*Pacing the floor, anxiously, muttering*): I'M SURE LITTLE WILLIE GREEN DIED OF WATER ON THE BRAIN! If only he could have been autopsied. What a sinful waste. Now we'll never know! I know what I'll do! I'll get Jake to bring the body up here and no one will know the difference. An inspiration! Positively the only solution! Why didn't I think of it before! Jake! Oh, Jake! Come here, please!

JAKE: Yass suh, doc, here I is.

DR. KELLY: Jake, how would you like to make $5.00?

JAKE: Who I gotta kill?

DR. KELLY: You won't have to kill anybody, Jake. Just run a very important errand for me and promise not to tell a soul.

JAKE: O.K., sounds good. What I gotta do?

DR. KELLY: Jake, do you remember little Willie Green?

JAKE: Yessuh, I owes him 50¢.

DR. KELLY: Well, Jake, Willie Green died this morning and was buried this afternoon. I want you to go to the cemetery and bring the body here.

JAKE: I just remembered—I forgot sumpin.

DR. KELLY: What did you forget?

JAKE: I forgot to stay home while I was there. (*Starts to go.*)

DR. KELLY (*Grabs him—pulls him to center stage and talks confidentially*): Jake, if you do a good job I'll not only give you the $5.00 but I'll throw in a gallon of gin.

JAKE: I'm your man!

DR. KELLY: OK, Jake, here's a big canvas bag. You bring him back in that. Do you know how to get to the cemetery?

JAKE: No suh—I ain't got no business in no cemetery. Sho' don't.

DR. KELLEY: OK, Jake, when you leave the house, turn left. Keep walking until you come to a fork in the road.

JAKE: Who lost de fork?

DR. KELLY: No, Jake—two roads—one goes this way and the others goes that way. I want you to take up the road to the right.

JAKE (*Throws bag at Doctor*): How de Hell I gonna do dat? I cain't TAKE UP NO ROAD!

DR. KELLY: No, Jake, you don't understand—you WALK up the road.

JAKE: Gimme the bag.

DR. KELLY: Then you'll come to the river. You'll see a rowboat there. Untie the boat and PULL UP the river!

JAKE (*Throws bag*): I cain't pull up no river!

DR. KELLY: No, no, no, Jake—you ROW up the river.

JAKE: OK, gimme the bag.

DR. KELLY: When you get to the other side you'll see a high stone wall.

JAKE: The Plenny tenchery.

DR. KELLY: No, Jake, the cemetery wall.

JAKE (*Throws bag*): I ain't got no business round no cemetery.

DR. KELLY: Jake, remember the $5.00.

JAKE: I don't need no $5.00.

DR. KELLY: Don't forget the gin!

JAKE: Gimme the bag!

DR. KELLY: Now when you walk over to the wall you'll see a tall ladder lying there. You put the ladder to the wall, climb up to the top and . . .

JAKE (*Throws bag*): Yeah, and some son of a gun yanks dat ladder away and there I'll be!

DR. KELLY: No one will be there to bother you. They're all dead.

JAKE: Dat's why I ain't goin!

DR. KELLY: Remember the $5.00.

JAKE: Nemind the $5.00.

DR. KELLY: The gin?

JAKE: Gimme the bag!

DR. KELLY: Now, once you get into the cemetery, you walk *past* two vaults on your RIGHT. The third one, you go in. Remove the lid from the first coffin. Feel the face. That's an old man with a long beard. That's not the man we want.

JAKE: Dat ain't de man we want.

DR. KELLY: Replace the lid, then check the next coffin. That's a lady with long hair . . .

JAKE: Dat ain't de man we want.

DR. KELLY: In the third coffin is little Willie Green . . .

JAKE (*Throws bag*): Take de bag. Just about dat time Willie gwine rise up and say, "Gimme dat 50¢ you owe me, boy." I ain't goin.

DR. KELLY: Remember the $5.00.

JAKE: Done told ya, don't need no $5.00.

DR. KELLY: Don't forget the gin!

JAKE: Gimme de bag.

DR. KELLY: OK now, you hurry and bring him up here and you'll get the gallon of gin and $5.00 too. (*Jake exits. Doctor paces a little more in self-satisfaction.*) I'd better go make preparations for the autopsy. (*Exits.*)

CURTAIN

(*Enter Charlie in front of curtain.*)

CHARLIE (*Thinking aloud*): I don't know how we can do it, but Kitty and I want to get married. Her father won't give his consent so we must elope. I've got to come up with a plan tonight or she may be too frightened to do it. (*Exits.*)

CURTAIN

(*Jake is onstage with a still form stretched out on the operating table.*)

JAKE: Doc—oh, Doc! I'm back.

DR. KELLY (*Enters. Shows elated surprise.*) My, that was fast work, Jake. You stay here now and keep an eye on him and I'll be right back to pay you. (*Exits.*)

JAKE (*Almost panics when the "corpse" sits up and turns out to be Charlie*): How'd *you* get in dat bag?

CHARLIE: Remember when you stopped to rest at the foot of the hill? Well, I took Willie out and I got in.

JAKE: You mean you let me carry you all the way up that hill? I'm gonna tell the Doc.

CHARLIE: No, Jake. Kitty and I plan to elope tonight. It was the only way I could safely enter the house. Now you've got to help us.

JAKE: How can I do dat?

CHARLIE: You can lie on the table until we get back.

JAKE: No suh—he's gonna do a cuttin' job on de corpse. I ain't gonna be no corpse.

CHARLIE: He won't autopsy until tomorrow.

JAKE: Well, OK. But what if something goes wrong?

CHARLIE: I won't be far away. You just yell out, "Over the river, Charlie," and I'll be RIGHT HERE. (*Exits as Jake lies down.*)

DR. KELLY (*Offstage. Yells*): This is what I'll use to cut out his diaphragm. (*Throws a carpenter's hand saw onto the stage.*)

JAKE (*Sits up*): Charlie! "Over the river, Charlie!"

CHARLIE (*Enters quickly*): What is it, Jake?

JAKE (*Pointing to the saw*): DAT's what he's gonna use to cut out my fryin' pan.

CHARLIE: Jake, I told you. He won't do anything until tomorrow. Do be quiet! (*Exits.*)

DR. KELLY (*Offstage*): This is my scalpel. (*He throws a big butcher knife on the stage.*)

JAKE: Charlie! "Over the river, Charlie!"

CHARLIE (*Reenters*): *Now* what?

JAKE (*Points at the knife*): He says he gonna SCALP HELL outta me!

CHARLIE: Not until tomorrow. Jake, be *quiet!* (*He exits on one side as Dr. Kelly enters on the other.*)

DR. KELLY: Aha—alone at last! (*He lifts the cover from the face and jumps back in surprise.*) I do believe half the proof is right here, right now, that I was right. The corpse is turning black already! Dear me! This means I can't wait till tomorrow. Let's see, I guess I'll start at this end.

(*Indicates the head. The doctor turns around and bends over to pick up a tool. As he does, Jake hastily switches ends. The doctor raises up cover and sees the feet where the head had been seconds before.*) Dear me! I've worried so much over this I'm afraid I'm losing my mind. I could have sworn the head was *here* a moment ago. Oh, well. I can work on his feet first, it really doesn't matter. (*He turns, bends over to exchange a tool, and Jake switches ends again. Doctor see that the feet are gone and the head is back. He walks toward the footlights.*) Something is very strange here. (*Charlie and Kitty come onstage.*)

KITTY (*Hugs father*): Oh, Daddy, Charlie and I just got married.

DR. KELLY: Well, since it's already done, I'll give you my blessing. (*He takes their right hands, holds them high over his head.*) May your first year be happiness and your second year joy . . .

JAKE (*Jumps up behind them*): . . . And the third year a girl, and the fourth a boy.

APPENDIX E

A Glossary of Pitchmen's Terms

AL-A-GA-ZAM: Hailing sign of pitchmen

BALLY or BALLY-ACT: Ballyhoo or attraction used to draw a crowd

BLOCKS: Watches

BLOOMERS: Poor business

BLOW-OFF: High-pressure selling used to liquidate stock before moving on

BLUE ONE: Poor business

BURR: Expenses

CAPPER: A confederate or shill

CARRY THE BANNER: To sleep in a park

CHOPPED GRASS: Herb medicines

CHUMP: Sucker

CLOSED TOWN: One in which pitchmen are refused a license

COCONUTS: Money

CORN PUNK or CORN SLUM: Any corn cure

EPPICE: Nothing or no good

FIXED: Ready for work, with the implication of buying off the police

FLASH: Flashy display of merchandise

FLEA POWDER: Powdered herbs

FLUKUM: Nickelplate ware; any liquid concoction

FUZZ: The police; a policeman

GASOLINE BILL BAKER: Stock name for any editor of the pitchmen's department in *The Billboard*

GILL: Customer; sucker

GIMMICK: Secret operating technique

GLIMS: Eyeglasses

GOOGS: Eyeglasses

GREASE: Salve

GRIFTER: A concessionaire operating various games of chance

GRINDER: Medical "lecturer"

GRIND JOINT: A "museum" or other place where lectures are given continuously

GUMMY: Glue

HICK: Sucker

HOME GUARD: Pitchmen who work only in their home cities

HOOPS: Rings

HOT SPOT: Excellent business location

JAMB: High-pressure tactics; any form of illegitimate selling

JOHNNY-COME-LATELY: A novice pitchman

KEISTER: A satchel which opens out to form a display case

LEARY: Damaged merchandise

LONG CON: Slow, deliberate persuasion

LOT LICE: Natives who arrive early and stay late without spending

NUT: Expenses

OPEN TOWN: One in which pitchmen may work after payment of a license fee

PASTE: Razor-strop dressing

PIPE: A letter, especially one to the pitchmen's department in *The Billboard*

PITCH: Sales talk to the crowd

PLUM: A good date

PUSH: Large crowd

READER: License to peddle

REDLIGHTED: Fired

RED ONE: Good business

RUBE: Sucker

SHILL: Confederate

SHIV: Knife or razor

SHORT CON: Brief, aggressive pitch or spiel

SIMP: Sucker

SLOUGH: To stop work for the day

SLUM: Cheap merchandise or prizes

SPIEL: A pitch

SQUAWKER: Complaining customer

STICK: A shill or confederate; a fountain pen

TIP: Prospects; a crowd; especially a small crowd

TRAILER: One who trails a show selling refreshments; especially one who does not pay for the privilege

TURN THE TIP: To activate a crowd to buy

VELVET: Profit

NOTES

Chapter 1

1. For a discussion of the European mountebank, see Grete de Francesco, *The Power of the Charlatan* (New Haven: Yale University Press, 1939), pp. 73–98.

2. Thomas Coryat, quoted in Samuel McKechnie, *Popular Entertainments Through the Ages* (London: Sampson Low, Marston and Co., Ltd., n.d.), pp. 56–57.

3. For a collection of English pitches, see *The Harangues, or Speeches, of Several Celebrated Quack-Doctors in Town and Country* (London, 1762).

4. Thomas Holcroft, quoted in C. J. S. Thompson, *The Quacks of Old London* (London: Brentano's Ltd., 1928), p. 75.

5. de Francesco, p. 80.

6. McKechnie, p. 58.

7. Thomas Coryat, quoted in *Ibid.*, p. 57.

8. *New York Mercury*, September 17, 1753.

9. William Smith, *The History of the Province of New-York . . . to the Year M. DCC. XXXII* (London, 1757), p. 212.

10. For a study of early American patent medicines, see James Harvey Young, *The Toadstool Millionaires; A Social History of Patent Medicines in America Before Federal Regulation* (Princeton, N.J., Princeton University Press, 1961).

11. For discussions of early American medical education, see Joseph F. Kett, *The Formation of the American Medical Profession* (New Haven: Yale University Press, 1968), and Henry B. Shafer, *The American Medical Profession, 1783 to 1850* (New York: Columbia University Press, 1936).

12. David L. Cowen, "Colonial Laws Pertaining to Pharmacy," *Journal of the American Pharmaceutical Association*, December 1934, pp. 1241–1242.

13. Quoted in Richardson Wright, *Hawkers and Walkers in Early America* (New York: Frederick Ungar Publishing Co., 1965), pp. 199–200.

14. *Massachusetts Spy,* September 5, 1771.

15. Isaac J. Greenwood, *The Circus, Its Origins and Growth Prior to 1835* (New York: The Dunlap Society, 1898), pp. 65–66.

16. Madge E. Pickard and R. Carlyle Buley, *The Midwest Pioneer, His Ills, Cures, and Doctors* (New York: Henry Schuman, 1946), p. 271; Allan Nevins, *John D. Rockefeller* (New York: Charles Scribner's Sons, 1941), I, 37–38; Arrell M. Gibson, "Medicine Show," *American West,* 1967, p. 35.

17. James Harvey Young, "American Medical Quackery in the Age of the Common Man," *Mississippi Valley Historical Review,* March 1961, p. 584.

18. *Warren County Leader* (Iowa), June 15, 1871, in *The Palimpsest,* June 1969, p. 368.

19. P. T. Barnum, *Struggles and Triumphs* (Buffalo, N.Y.: The Courier Co., 1889), p. 185.

20. In Pickard and Buley, pp. 286–287.

21. In Adelaide Hechtlinger, *The Great Patent Medicine Era* (New York: Grosset and Dunlap, Inc., 1970), p. 56.

22. Advertisement in the Bella C. Landauer Collection of the New-York Historical Society.

23. In Hechtlinger, p. 56; *The Palimpsest,* June 1969, p. 318.

24. Young, "American Medical Quackery in the Age of the Common Man," p. 586.

25. James Harvey Young, "The Patent Medicine Almanac," *Wisconsin Magazine of History,* Spring 1962, pp. 159–163; Dorothea D. Reeves, "Come All for the Cure-all," *Harvard Library Bulletin,* 1967, pp. 253–272; William J. Petersen, "Patent Medicine Advertising Cards," *The Palimpsest,* June 1969, pp. 317–331.

26. Letter from Milton Bartok, February 9, 1970.

27. Interview, Booth's Corner, Pennsylvania, July 1970; for a study of the pitchman and radio and television advertising, see Long John Nebel, "The Pitchman," *Harper's,* May 1961, pp. 50–54.

Chapter 2

1. Dr. Bullywat, "When High Pitchmen Had Brains," unidentified clipping in a scrapbook, made by a medicine showman, in the collection of William Helfand. The scrapbook, which may have been assembled by a showman who styled himself The Great Cummings and Diamond Bill Cummings Ph.D., contains about eighty pages of clippings, labels flyers, and other medicine show items, most of which appear to date from the first quarter of the twentieth century. Cited hereafter as Helfand Scrapbook.

2. Thomas P. Kelley, Jr., *The Fabulous Kelley* (Richmond Hill, Ontario: Simon and Schuster of Canada, Ltd., 1968), pp. 14–15, 72–73.

3. Ralph and Richard Rinzler (eds.), Notes to *Old-Time Music at Clarence Ashley's*, Folkways Records Album FA2355, p. 2. Ashley was an entertainer with various medicine shows, notably Doc Hower's Mokiton Tonic show, from about 1916 to 1943.

4. Violet McNeal, *Four White Horses and a Brass Band* (Garden City, N.Y.: Doubleday and Co., Inc., 1947), p. 43.

5. *Ibid.*, pp. 43–44.

6. *Ibid.*, p. 44.

7. Undated clipping from *Advertising World*, Helfand Scrapbook.

8. *Ibid.*

9. N. T. Oliver (as told to Wesley Stout), "Alagazam, The Story of Pitchmen, High and Low," *Saturday Evening Post*, October 19, 1929, p. 76; Sid Sidenberg, "Pitchdom Forty Years Ago and Today," in *Amusement Business*, December 31, 1969, p. 153; "Picturesque Medicine Shows Combined Entertainment with Salesmanship," *Missouri Historical Review*, 1951, p. 375.

10. Rinzler, p. 2.

11. Stewart H. Holbrook, *The Golden Age of Quackery* (New York: The Macmillan Company, 1959), p. 198.

12. Interview with Mr. and Mrs. Milton Bartok, Fairfax, Virginia, April 1970. Cited hereafter as Bartok Interview.

13. Rinzler, p. 2; Sidenberg, p. 153.

14. *Ibid.*; Arthur H. Lewis, *Carnival* (New York: Trident Press, 1970), p. 138.

15. Bartok Interview.

16. Sidenberg, p. 153.

17. Dr. Bullywat, Helfand Scrapbook; McNeal, p. 101.

18. Winifred Johnston, "Medicine Show," *Southwest Review*, Summer 1936, p. 395; Gerald Carson, *One for a Man, Two for a Horse* (Garden City, N.Y.: Doubleday and Co., 1961), p. 68; Pat Dalton, letter to "Pipes for Pitchmen," *The Billboard*, October 2, 1920, p. 66; N. T. Oliver (as told to Wesley Stout), "Med Show," *Saturday Evening Post*, September 14, 1929, p. 169; Rinzler, p. 2.

19. McNeal, pp. 150–154.

20. Thomas J. LeBlanc, "The Medicine Show," *American Mercury*, June 1925, p. 236; Holbrook, p. 199; McNeal, pp. 69–70; Kelley, pp. 109–110.

21. Bartok Interview.

22. McNeal, pp. 64–65; Holbrook, pp. 202–203; George Jean Nathan, "The Medicine Man," *Harper's Weekly*, September 9, 1911, p. 24.

23. Bartok Interview.

24. "Rolling Ten Pins?" unidentified clipping, Helfand Scrapbook.

25. Bartok Interview.

26. *Ibid;* McNeal, p. 155.

27. Bartok Interview.

28. McNeal, p. 198.

29. Advertisements, *The Billboard*, October 2, 1920, pp. 66–67; O. Henry, "Jeff Peters As a Personal Magnet," in *The Gentle Grafter* (New York: Doubleday, Page and Co., 1916), p. 22; Robert Lewis Taylor, "Talker" *The New Yorker*, April 19, 1958, pp. 48–49.

30. Advertisement, Herb Remedy Company, Blair, Nebraska, Helfand Scrapbook.

31. Letter, H. E. Christiansen to William L. Cummings, June 16, 1914, Helfand Scrapbook.

32. McNeal, pp. 63–64; W. A. S. Douglas, "Pitch Doctors," *American Mercury*, February 1927, p. 225.

33. *Ibid.*

34. Interview with Flo St. John, Fairfax, Virginia, April 1970. Cited hereafter as St. John Interview.

35. Douglas, p. 225; McNeal, p. 38.

36. William P. Burt, "Back Stage with a Medicine Show Fifty Years Ago," *Colorado Magazine*, July 1942, p. 136.

37. Flyer, Quillaia Soap, Helfand Scrapbook.

38. McNeal, p. 164.

39. *Ibid.*

40. Douglas, p. 225.

41. Pickard and Buley, pp. 278–79.

42. *Life and Scenes Among the Kickapoo Indians* (New Haven: Healy and Bigelow, n.d.), p. 102. University of Oklahoma Library.

43. Douglas Gilbert, *American Vaudeville* (New York: Dover Publications, Inc., 1963), p. 215; Oliver, "Med Show," p. 169.

44. Holbrook, p. 209.

45. Dr. Bullywat, "When High Pitchmen Had Brains"; Oliver, "Med Show," p. 174.

46. Dr. Bullywat, "When High Pitchmen Had Brains"; C. F. Fowler, "The Art of Selling Medical Goods by Exhibition," unidentified clipping, Helfand Scrapbook.

47. Oliver, "Med Show," p. 173.

48. McNeal, pp. 62–63.

49. Kelley, p. 19.

50. Lewis Atherton, *Main Street on the Middle Border* (Bloomington: Indiana University Press, 1954), p. 160.

51. Clipping, New York *World,* April 9, 1916, Helfand Scrapbook. For material on the life and career of "Painless" Parker, see Richard Donovan and Dwight Whitney, "Last of America's Tooth Plumbers," *Collier's,* January 5, 12, 19, 1952. Parker, like many other dental parlor operators, began his career as a dental pitchman.

52. Interview with Milton Lomax, June 1970, Stony Brook, New York.

53. Donovan and Whitney, January 12, 1952, p. 43.

54. Oliver, "Med Show," p. 13; Carson, p. 61; McNeal, p. 68.

55. Eric Jameson, *The Natural History of Quackery* (London: Michael Joseph, 1961), p. 184.

56. Harlowe R. Hoyt, *Town Hall Tonight* (New York: Bramhall House, 1955), pp. 245–246.

57. Letter, Donald McKay to William McKay, October 24, 1880, William McKay Papers, Unatilla County Library, Pendleton, Oregon.

58. Oliver, "Alagazam," p. 76; Lewis, p. 140.

59. "The Passing of Big Foot Wallace," *The Billboard,* March 31, 1917, in *Amusement Business,* December 31, 1969, p. 153.

60. John C. Duval, *The Adventures of Big-Foot Wallace, the Texas Ranger and Hunter,* ed. by Mabel Major and Rebecca Smith Lee (Lincoln: University of Nebraska Press, 1966).

61. *Ibid.,* xiii–xxix; E. A. Botkin (ed.), *A Treasury of American Folklore* (New York: Crown Publishers, 1949), pp. 133, 157–159; "William Alexander Anderson Wallace," *Dictionary of American Biography,* XIX, 377–378.

62. "The Passing of Big Foot Wallace," p. 153.

63. Dr. Bullywat, "When High Pitchmen Had Brains."

64. J. I. Lighthall, *The Indian Household Medicine Guide* (Peoria, Illinois, n.p., 1883), pp. 136–137; mail diagnosis sheet, New England Medical Institute, Boston, Massachusetts, n.p., n.d., collection of the National Library of Medicine, Bethesda, Maryland; "Fake Doctoring by Mail," unidentified clipping, Helfand Scrapbook.

65. Oliver, "Med Show," p. 169.

66. "Fake Doctoring by Mail."

67. Bartok Interview; Oliver, "Alagazam," p. 76.

68. McNeal, p. 122.

69. Oliver, "Alagazam," p. 76; Douglas, p. 223.

70. *Ibid.*

71. Oliver, "Med Show," p. 169; Holbrook, pp. 198–199; Jim Tully, "The Giver of Life," *American Mercury*, June 1928, p. 156; Holbrook, p. 199.

72. Kelley, p. 182.

73. Douglas, p. 223.

74. Bartok Interview.

75. *Ibid.*

76. Oliver, "Alagazam," p. 76; Douglas, pp. 223–224.

77. *Ibid.*, p. 224.

78. Bartok Intervew.

79. McNeal, p. 123.

80. *Ibid.*, pp. 125–126.

81. Cf. Rollin Lynde Hartt, *The People at Play* (Boston: Houghton Mifflin Company, 1909), pp. 85–112.

82. Holbrook, pp. 77–78, 80.

83. *Ibid.*, p. 83.

84. Jameson, p. 97; Holbrook, p. 76; McNeal, p. 139.

85. Broadside, New York Museum of Anatomy, New-York Historical Society.

86. Holbrook, pp. 76–77.

87. Quoted in Robert Soucey, "The Egregious Quacks," *MD*, August 1971, p. 99.

88. Flyer, *The Spieler*, Helfand Scrapbook.

89. Advertisement, Silver Cloud, Helfand Scrapbook.

Chapter 3

1. Charles T. Hunt, Sr. (as told to John C. Cloutman), *The Story of Mr. Circus* (Rochester, N.H.: The Record Press, 1954), pp. 20–21, 49, 57, 68.

2. Interview with Bobby Snyder, Fairfax, Virginia, April 1970. Cited hereafter as Snyder Interview; Lewis, p. 138; Kelley, p. 176.

3. Snyder Interview. Interview with Mr. and Mrs. Bob Styer, Reading, Pennsylvania, July 1970; cited hereafter as Styer Interview.

4. Bartok Interview.

5. *Ibid.*

6. Letter, Donald McKay to William McKay, October 24, 1880; Gilbert, p. 215; Holbrook, p. 205; Kelley, pp. 182, 7; Donovan and Whitney, p. 7.

7. Oliver, pp. 12–13, 169, 173; Gilbert, pp. 215–218; clipping, "The Sturdy House of Hamlin," Chicago *Tribune*, July 21, 1931, Chicago Historical Society; Frank Joslyn Baum and Russel P. McFall, *To Please a Child* (Chicago: Reilly and Lee Co., 1961), pp. 11–12.

8. Bartok Interview.

9. Kelley, p. 101.

10. *Ibid*, pp. 101–102.

11. Harry Leon Wilson, *Professor, How Could You!* (New York: Cosmopolitan Book Corporation, 1924), p. 121.

12. Snyder Interview; Bartok Interview; LeBlanc, p. 235.

13. St. John Interview.

14. Lewis, p. 139.

15. Bartok Interview.

16. Letter from Joseph L. Barr, August 26, 1969.

17. Rinzler, p. 2; Styer Interview; Kelley, p. 7.

18. *Ibid*.

19. *Ibid.*, p. 95.

20. Letter, F. E. Karn to W. L. Cummings, March 10, 1903, Helfand Scrapbook.

21. Sidenberg, p. 153; letter from Anna Mae Noell, June 26, 1970; Kelley, p. 63.

22. Bartok Interview; "Medicine Show Notes," undated clipping from *The Billboard,* Helfand Scrapbook; Kelley, p. 15.

23. "Medicine Show Notes."

24. Oregon Indian Medicine Company, board contract form, Helfand Scrapbook.

25. "Manager of Public, or Opera Hall," contract form, Helfand Scrapbook; "Hall or Lot Contract," Helfand Scrapbook.

26. "East Indian Remedy Company," questionnaire, Townsend Walsh Collection, Research Library of the Performing Arts, Lincoln Center.

27. "Hall or Lot Contract."

28. Bartok Interview; Snyder Interview; Kelley, pp. 74, 101.

29. Cf. Atherton, pp. 136–142.

30. Lomax Interview.

31. Kelley, p. 50.

32. Snyder Interview.

33. Graydon Laverne Freeman, *The Medicine Showman* (Watkins Glen, N.Y.: Century House, 1957), p. 5; Styer Interview.

34. F. J. Clifford, "The Medicine Show," *Frontier Times,* December 1930, p. 95.

35. Burt, p. 129.

36. Snyder Interview; Kelly p. 170.

37. Cummings, "One Phase of the Medicine Show Business."

38. Bartok Interview.

39. *Ibid.*

40. *Ibid.;* Snyder Interview; cf., Irving Zeidman, *The American Burlesque Show* (New York: Hawthorn Books, Inc., 1967), pp. 197–200.

41. Snyder Interview.

42. Styer Interview; Rinzler, p. 2.

43. Styer Interview; interview with Bill Smith, New York City, February 1972. Cited hereafter as Smith Interview.

44. Clifford, p. 95.

45. *Ibid.*, p. 85; Rinzler, p. 2; Smith Interview.

46. Tully, p. 157; Bartok Interview; McNeal, pp. 100–106.

47. Holbrook, p. 187.

48. Holtman, p. 231.

49. Johnston, p. 392.

50. Cummings, "One Phase of the Medicine Business."

51. Photographs of Webb's laboratory by Russell Lee, Pine Bluff, Arkansas, September 1938, Prints and Photographs Division, Library of Congress.

52. Interview with Harve Hamilton by James Harvey Young, Girard, Illinois, 1958; trade card, the Clifton Remedy Company, Helfand Scrapbook.

53. Quoted in Thompson, p. 142.

54. Oliver, "Alagazam," p. 76.

55. "A Telegraph Cipher," circular, German Medicine Company, Helfand Scrapbook; "Telegraph Code," circular, German Medicine Company, Helfand Scrapbook.

56. *Ibid.*

57. Price list, German Medicine Company, Helfand Scrapbook.

58. *Ibid.*

59. "Billing Like a Circus," *The Billboard*, September 1, 1896, in *Amusement Business*, December 31, 1969, p. 139.

60. *The Wild West* (Fort Worth: Amon Carter Museum of Western Art, 1970), p. 96; A. Morton Smith, "Forty Years of Circus Advertising," in *Amusement Business*, December 31, 1969, p. 163.

61. Hunt, pp. 78, 189–190.

62. Price list, German Medicine Company.

63. Stock showbill, German Medicine Company, Helfand Scrapbook.

64. *Ibid.*

65. Price List, German Medicine Company.

Chapter 4

1. Oliver, "Med Show," p. 174.

2. William Lee Provol, *The Pack Peddler* (Greenville, Pa.: The Beaver Printing Company, 1933), p. 107.

3. Nathan, p. 24.

4. Oliver, "Med Show," p. 173.

5. Bartok Interview.

6. Holbrook, p. 197.

7. Carson, p. 64.

8. Hoyt, pp. 246–247.

9. McNeal, pp. 55–56.

10. Shaker Medicine Company labels, pamphlets, and circulars, Bella C. Landauer Collection.

11. Harry D. Piercy, *Shaker Medicine,* reprinted from *Selected Papers,* Shaker Historical Society, October 1957, p. 20.

12. Burt, pp. 134–136.

13. "The Sturdy House of Hamlin"; Burt, p. 128; Hoyt, pp. 248–251.

14. Arthur J. Cramp, *Nostrums and Quackery* (3 vols.; Chicago: American Medical Association, 1912–1936), II, p. 596.

15. *Ibid.,* I, p. 600.

16. Labels, Bella C. Landauer Collection; Oliver, "Med Show," p. 174.

17. Burt, p. 128; Oliver, "Med Show," p. 174.

18. Six Hamlin songsters bearing various titles are in the Brown University Library, Providence, Rhode Island.

19. *Hamlin's Wizard Oil, the Book of Songs* (Chicago: Hamlin's Wizard Oil Co., n.d.). Bella C. Landauer Collection.

20. Oliver, "Med Show," p. 174.

21. Burt, p. 128.

22. *Ibid.*

23. *Ibid.*

24. *Ibid.*

25. Oliver, "Alagazam," p. 79; letter from Joseph L. Barr, August 26, 1969.

26. Hoyt, pp. 248–251.

27. Oliver, "Med Show," p. 174.

28. Burt, p. 131.

29. Circular, Modern Miracles, Helfand Scrapbook.

30. Burt, pp. 132–133.

31. William R. Cagle, "James Whitcomb Riley: Notes on the Early Years," *Manuscripts,* Spring 1965, p. 5.

32. Marcus Dickey, *The Youth of James Whitcomb Riley* (Indianapolis: The Bobbs-Merrill Co., 1919), pp. 200–201; Richard Crowder, *Those Innocent Years* (Indianapolis: The Bobbs-Merrill Co., 1957), p. 68.

33. Dickey, pp. 199–200.

34. *Ibid.,* pp. 198–199.

35. *Ibid.,* p. 201.

Chapter 5

1. Oliver, "Med Show," p. 12. Unless otherwise noted, material on the early careers of Healy and Bigelow is taken from Oliver's two articles, "Med Show" and "Alagazam."

2. Cramp, I, p. 600; Holbrook, p. 214.

3. Oliver, "Alagazam," p. 79.

4. Oliver, "Med Show," p. 169.

5. *Life and Scenes Among the Kickapoo Indians,* p. 79; Nathan, p. 132; *Kickapoo Indian Dream Book* (New Haven: Kickapoo Indian Medicine Company, n.d.), p. 1, Townsend Walsh Collection.

6. David Adams, "When the Kickapoos Cared for New Haven's Ills," pp. 31–32, manuscript copy of a newspaper article from the New Haven *Register,* January 16, 1921. New Haven Colony Historical Society; Holbrook, p. 213.

7. N. T. Oliver, *The Priceless Recipes* (Chicago: Laird and Lee, 1900), p. 44.

8. McNeal, p. 53.

9. Adams, p. 30; Holbrook, pp. 210, 214–215.

10. Adams, p. 31.

11. *Life and Scenes Among the Kickapoo Indians,* pp. 72–73.

12. *Ibid.*

13. For information on the use of the Indian symbol by patent medicine manufacturers, see James Harvey Young, "Patent Medicines and Indians," *Emory University Quarterly,* Summer 1961, pp. 86–92, and Carson, pp. 23–29.

14. Cf. Young, "Patent Medicines and Indians," pp. 86–88.

15. Pickard and Buley, pp. 36–37.

16. *Ibid.,* pp. 45, 72–73.

17. Circular, Oregon Indian Medicine Company, Bella C. Landauer Collection.

18. *Enquire Within for Many Useful Facts Relating to Your Health and Happiness* (New Haven: The Kickapoo Indians, n.d.), p. 8, Bella C. Landauer Collection.

19. Miscellaneous Kickapoo publications in the Bella C. Landauer Collection, the Townsend Walsh Collection, the University of Oklahoma Library, and the collection of William Helfand.

20. Cf. James Harvey Young, "The Patent Medicine Almanac," pp. 159–164.

21. *The Kickapoo Indians and Their Medicine Men* (New York: Great American Engraving and Printing Co., n.d.), p. 1, Bella C. Landauer Collection.

22. *Life and Scenes Among the Kickapoo Indians,* p. 2.

23. *First Time of Everything* (New Haven: Kickapoo Indian Medicine Company, n.d.), rear cover, Bella C. Landauer Collection.

24. *Kickapoo Indians: Life and Scenes Among the Indians* (New Haven: Kickapoo Indian Medicine Company, n.d.), p. 1, Townsend Walsh Collection.

25. *Ibid.* p. 7ff.; N. T. Oliver, *Mexican Bill, the Cowboy Detective* (Chicago: Eagle Publishing Company, 1888). A number of Oliver's mysteries and other writings are in the collection of the Library of Congress, Washington, D.C.

26. *Enquire Within,* p. 8.

27. "Sagwa's Surprising Story: How Texas Charlie's Life Was Saved by the Indians," *Kickapoo Indian Life and Scenes* (n.p., n.d.), p. 26, Townsend Walsh Collection.

28. Mark Twain, quoted in Laurence Hutton, *Curiosities of the American Stage* (New York: Harper & Brothers, 1891), p. 17.

Chapter 6

1. G. C. D. Odell, *Annals of the New York Stage* (New York: Columbia University Press, 1927), I, p. 131.

2. New York *Post,* October 30, 1827.

3. *Life and Scenes Among the Kickapoo Indians,* p. 78.

4. *Ibid.*

5. Oliver, "Med Show," p. 169.

6. Gibson, p. 76; Holbrook, p. 209; Oliver, "Med Show," p. 173.

7. Gibson, p. 76.

8. Holbrook, p. 210; Oliver, "Med Show," p. 173; Kelley, p. 145.

9. "The Kickapoo Reservation—Self-Supporting, Self-Respecting Kickapoos," *Kickapoo Indian Life and Scenes,* pp. 16–17.

10. *Life and Scenes Among the Kickapoo Indians*, p. 117.

11. *First Time of Everything*, inside rear cover.

12. Adams, p. 31.

13. Oliver, "Med Show," pp. 173–174.

14. Kickapoo advertisement, Bella C. Landauer Collection.

15. Carl Sandburg, *Always the Young Strangers* (New York: Harcourt, Brace and Company, 1953), p. 270.

16. Gay MacLaren, *Morally We Roll Along* (Boston: Little, Brown and Co., 1938), p. 31.

17. Holbrook, p. 212.

18. Oliver, "Med Show," p. 173.

19. *Ibid.*

20. Kickapoo circular, Harvard Theatre Collection.

21. *Ibid.*

22. Holbrook, pp. 212–213.

23. All information on the Albany performances is from the Townsend Walsh Scrapbook, Townsend Walsh Collection.

24. Oliver, "Med Show," p. 174; *The Indian,* n.d., n.p., Bella C. Landauer Collection; Adams, p. 31; Young, "Patent Medicines and Indians"; Carson, p. 64; *Life and Scenes Among the Kickapoo Indians,* p. 14.

25. Cummings, "One Phase of the Medicine Business," Helfand Scrapbook.

Chapter 7

1. *Life and Scenes Among the Kickapoo Indians,* p. 155.

2. Carson, p. 27.

3. Advertisements, Bella C. Landauer Collection and possession of the author.

4. Letter, Donald McKay to William McKay, October 24, 1880, William McKay Papers.

5. Letter W. F. Cody to William McKay, December 7 (year not given), William McKay Papers.

6. Letter, Donald McKay to William McKay, April 28, 1888, William KcKay Papers.

7. David Edstrom, "Medicine Men of the '80's," *Readers Digest,* June 1938, p. 71.

8. Will Rose, *The Vanishing Village* (New York: Citadel Press, 1963), p. 130.

9. Oliver, "Med Show," p. 173.

10. Dr. James M. Solomon, Jr., *Advice to Invalids,* n.p., n.d., p. 4, Bella C. Landauer Collection.

11. Freeman, p. 5; Provol, pp. 106–107.

12. Wilson, p. 125.

13. *Ibid.*, p. 127.

14. Edwin Eastman, *Captured and Branded by the Camanche [sic] Indians in the Year 1860*, n.p., n.d., Bella C. Landauer Collection; Young, "Patent Medicines and Indians," pp. 89–90.

15. Rose, p. 136.

16. Wilson, p. 129; Robert Lewis Taylor, *A Journey to Matecumbe* (New York: Avon Books, 1961), pp. 72–73; Oliver, "Med Show," p. 173.

17. Joe Sappington, "The Passing of the Medicine Show," *Frontier Times*, February 1930, pp. 229–230; Edstrom, pp. 77–78.

18. Freeman, pp. 5–6.

19. Charles L. Pancoast, *Trail Blazers of Advertising* (New York: Frederick H. Hitchcock, 1926), p. 64.

20. Provol, p. 108.

21. Edstrom, p. 78.

22. Letter from William Ruesskamp, May 23, 1970; Cummings, "One Phase of the Medicine Business," Helfand Scrapbook.

23. Wilson, p. 130.

24. McNeal, pp. 102–104.

25. Advertising card, Helfand Scrapbook.

26. Form letter, Suter Remedy Company, Helfand Scrapbook.

27. Oregon Indian Medicine Company circular, Bella C. Landauer Collection.

Chapter 8

1. Material on the life of T. A. Edwards, unless otherwise noted, is taken from John Miller, *A Twentieth Century History of Erie County, Pennsylvania* (Chicago: Lewis Publishing Co., 1909), II, 627–628, and *Nelson's Biographical Dictionary and Historical Reference Book of Erie County, Pennsylvania* (Erie, Pa.: S. B. Nelson, 1896), p. 768.

2. A pay voucher made out to Edwards as a "United States Special Detective," dated May 28, 1863, and a certificate stating his duties, dated April 14, 1863, are in the National Archives, Washington, D. C. Letter from Keith Clark, January 11, 1971.

3. Keith A. Murray, *The Modocs and Their War* (Norman: University of Oklahoma Press, 1959), p. 199. An Oregon Indian Medicine Company publication supposedly written by McKay (*Indian Scout Life*, n.d., p. 1, Bella C. Landauer Collection) claims that his mother was a Nez Percé and his paternal grandmother an Iroquois.

4. Dee Brown, *Bury My Heart at Wounded Knee* (New York: Bantam Books, Inc., 1971), p. 233.

5. *Daring Donald McKay, or the Last War-Trail of the Modocs* (Chicago: Rounds Brothers, 1881), unnumbered page.

6. Letter, Donald McKay to William McKay, March 6, 1892, William McKay Papers.

7. Letter, Donald McKay to William McKay, April 28, 1888, William McKay Papers.

8. *Ibid.*

9. *Nelson's Biographical Dictionary,* p. 768.

10. Letter, Donald McKay to William McKay, November 7, 1890, William McKay Papers.

11. Letter, Donald McKay to William McKay, April 28, 1888, William McKay Papers.

12. Circular, Oregon Indian Medicine Company, Helfand Scrapbook.

13. Circular directed to showmen, Oregon Indian Medicine Company, Helfand Scrapbook.

14. Oregon Indian Medicine Company envelope, 1890, William McKay Papers.

15. Del Darling in Corry *Times-News,* July 9, 1961.

16. Circular, Oregon Indian Medicine Company, Helfand Scrapbook.

17. Cramp, II, 602.

18. Corry *Times-News,* July 9, 1961.

19. Oregon Indian Medicine Company envelope, 1890, William McKay Papers; Cummings, "One Phase of the Medicine Business," Helfand Scrapbook; circular, Oregon Indian Medicine Company, Helfand Scrapbook.

20. Circular, Oregon Indian Medicine Company, Bella C. Landauer Collection.

21. Guarantee, Oregon Indian Medicine Company, Helfand Scrapbook.

22. Price list, Oregon Indian Medicine Company, Helfand Scrapbook; an admission ticket from the Oregon Indian Medicine Company is in the Helfand Collection.

23. *Indian Scout Life,* inside front cover.

24. *Ibid.,* p. 2.

25. Circular, Modern Miracles, Helfand Scrapbook.

26. W. L. Cummings, "One Phase of the Medicine Business," Helfand Scrapbook.

27. Kelley, pp. 144–145.

28. Cummings, "One Phase of the Medicine Business," Helfand Scrapbook.

29. Oliver, "Alagazam," p. 79; a selection of advertising materials from the Iroquois Famous Indian Remedies Company of Harlem is in the Theatre Collection, Museum of the City of New York.

30. Oliver, "Med Show," p. 174.

31. *Ibid.*

32. Clipping, "Col. C. Bigelow," Helfand Scrapbook.

33. Cummings, "One Phase of the Medicine Business," Helfand Scrapbook; letter to W. H. Kelley, from the Kickapoo Indian Medicine Company, December 23, 1914, Helfand Scrapbook.

34. Adams, p. 31.

Chapter 9

1. Wright, p. 199.

2. Lewis, p. 140; Neil E. Schaffner with Vance Johnson, *The Fabulous Toby and Me* (Englewood Cliffs, N.J.: Prentice-Hall, Inc., 1968), pp. 13–14.

3. Sinclair Lewis, *Main Street* (New York: Harcourt, Brace & World, Inc., 1920), pp. 224–225.

4. *Ibid.*, p. 171.

5. Lomax Interview; Styer Interview.

6. Letter from Milton Bartok, February 9, 1970; Oliver, "Alagazam," p. 70.

7. Among the show business figures who worked in medicine shows were Houdini, Fred Stone, Charles Winninger, Fred Allen, the Weaver Brothers, Hal Skelly, Pig Meat Martin, Peg Leg Bates, Bob Crosby, Red Skelton, Joe Cook, Roy Acuff, Jimmie Rodgers, Tex Ritter, and Hank Williams. See Johnston, p. 394; Fred Stone, *Rolling Stone* (New York: McGraw-Hill Book Company, Inc., 1945), p. 58; Douglas, p. 222; Kelley, p. 184; Oliver, "Alagazam," pp. 79–80; Bartok Interview; Charles Winninger obituary, New York *Times*, January 29, 1969; Milbourne Christopher, *Houdini, The Untold Story* (New York: Pocket Books, 1970), pp. 26–27; Bill C. Malone, *Country Music U.S.A.* (Austin: University of Texas Press, 1968), p. 20.

8. W. L. Cummings, "One Phase of the Medicine Show Business," Helfand Scrapbook.

9. Clipping, "Wanted for the Becker Medicine Show," Helfand Scrapbook.

10. W. L. Cummings, "One Phase of the Medicine Show Business," Helfand Scrapbook.

11. Letter from Milton Bartok, February 9, 1970.

12. Snyder Interview.

13. Oliver, "Alagazam," p. 79.

14. For a discussion of comic stereotypes see Constance Rourke, *American Humor* (New York: Harcourt, Brace and Company, Inc., 1931).

15. Cf. William Lawrence Slout, *Theatre in a Tent* (Bowling Green, Ohio: Bowling Green University Popular Press, 1972), pp. 72–73.

16. Letter from Anna Mae Noell, August 12, 1972; Bartok Interview.

17. Snyder Interview.

18. For the relationship of other popular forms to *commedia dell' arte* see Ralph Allen, "Our Native Theatre: Honky-Tonk, Minstrel Shows, Burlesque," in Henry B. Williams (ed.), *The American Theatre: A Sum of Its Parts* (New York: Samuel French, Inc., 1971), pp. 280–281; and Richard Moody (ed.), *Dramas From the American Theatre, 1762–1909* (Cleveland: The World Publishing Company, 1966), p. 483.

19. Snyder Interview.

20. Styer Interview; St. John Interview.

21. For a discussion of the "nigger act" in burlesque, see Allen, pp. 281–282.

22. Styer Interview.

23. Letter from Bill Ruesskamp, August 6, 1970.

24. Claude Gamble, "The Medicine Show," manuscript sketch written for the Peoria *Star,* in the possession of Robert Gamble, Sea Cliff, New York.

25. Kelley, pp. 58, 71.

26. Lomax Interview.

27. Christopher, pp. 26–31; Kelley, p. 58.

28. McNeal, pp. 196–197.

29. *Ibid.,* 197.

30. LeBlanc, p. 236.

31. Letter from Anna Mae Noell, July 30, 1972.

32. Clifford, p. 93.

33. Barnum, pp. 65–66.

34. Ross, p. 137; Snyder Interview; letter from Anna Mae Noell, July 30, 1972.

35. W. L. Cummings, "One Phase of the Medicine Show Business," Helfand Scrapbook; letter from Anna Mae Noell, July 30, 1972.

36. Kelley, pp. 20–21.

37. Flyers, Modern Remedy Company and German Medicine Company, Helfand Scrapbook.

38. Cohn, p. 215.

39. Letter from Anna Mae Noell, July 30, 1972.

40. LeBlanc, p. 233; Cohn, p. 213.

41. Kelley, p. 52.

42. *Ibid.,* 119.

43. Letter from Anna Mae Noell, July 15, 1972.

44. Letter from Anna Mae Noell, no date.

45. *Ibid.*

46. Letter from Anna Mae Noell, July 15, 1972. The catalogue of a professional writer who catered to vaudeville artists, medicine show people, and other variety performers, lists about 35 traditional medicine show acts available at $3.00 each. Catalogue, "Uncle Cal," possession of the author.

47. Letter from Anna Mae Noell, July 30, 1972.

48. Kelley, p. 19.

49. Gilbert, p. 48.

50. Letter from Anna Mae Noell, June 15, 1972.

Chapter 10

1. For an extensive discussion of legislation, see Young, *The Toadstool Millionaires,* pp. 205–244.

2. Cramp, I. pp. 555–556.

3. Circular, C. I. Hood Company, Helfand Collection.

4. Letter, W. H. Suter to W. L. Cummings, September 19, 1916, Helfand Scrapbook.

5. "Of Interest to Medicine Men," *New York Clipper,* February 24, 1912, "More About the Richardson Bill," March 2, 1912: clipping, "'Patent Medicines' and Others," Helfand Scrapbook.

6. Holbrook, pp. 23–24.

7. Bartok Interview.

8. Kelley, p. 180.

9. Johnston, p. 396.

10. Snyder Interview.

11. Bartok Interview.

12. *Ibid.*

13. Johnston, p. 396.

14. For more detailed studies of LeBlanc's career, see Young, "The Hadacol Phenomenon," *Emory University Quarterly,* June 1951, pp. 72–86, and *The Medical Messiahs* (Princeton: Princeton University Press, 1967), pp. 316–332.

15. Pete Collins, *No People Like Show People* (London: Frederick Muller Ltd., 1957), p. 162.

16. Collins, pp. 155–183, provides an interesting firsthand account of life with the Caravan.

17. Bartok Interview.

18. Young, *The Medical Messiahs*, pp. 323–324.

19. David Nevin, "The Brass-Band Pitchman and His Million-Dollar Elixer," *True*, March 1962, p. 18.

20. Collins, p. 162.

21. Newspaper advertisement, Hadacol Caravan Show, Atlanta *Journal*, August 21, 1951, James Harvey Young Collection.

22. Nevin, pp. 16–17.

23. Flyer, Hadacol Caravan Show, James Harvey Young Collection.

24. The description of the Atlanta show is based on manuscript notes made at the performance by James Harvey Young and on articles which appeared in the Atlanta *Constitution*, August 19, 1951 and August 24, 1951.

25. Smith Interview; Bartok Interview; letter from Milton Bartok, February 9, 1970.

26. Letter from Bill Sachs, June 1, 1970.

27. Letter from Milton Bartok, February 9, 1970.

28. Nebel, p. 50.

29. E. E. Cummings, *Him* (New York: Liveright Publishing Company, 1927), pp. 44–45.

BIBLIOGRAPHY

Books

Atherton, Lewis. *Main Street on the Middle Border*. Bloomington: Indiana University Press, 1954.

Barnum, P. T. *Struggles and Triumphs*. Buffalo: The Courier
Co., 1889.

Baum, Frank Joslyn, and McFall, Russel P. *To Please a Child*.
Chicago: Reilly and Lee, 1961.

Botkin, E. A., ed. *A Treasury of American Folklore*. New York:
Crown Publishers, 1949.

Brown, Dee. *Bury My Heart at Wounded Knee*. New York: Bantam
Books, Inc., 1971.

Carson, Gerald. *One for a Man, Two for a Horse*. Garden City,
N.Y.: Doubleday & Co., Inc., 1961.

Christopher, Milbourne. *Houdini, The Untold Story*. New York:
Pocket Books, 1970.

Collins, Pete. *No People Like Show People*. London: Frederick
Muller, Ltd., 1957.

Cramp, Arthur J. *Nostrums and Quackery*. 3 vols. Chicago: American Medical Association, 1912–1936.

Crowder, Richard. *Those Innocent Years*. Indianapolis: The Bobbs-
Merrill Co., 1957.

Cummings, E. E. *Him*. New York: Liveright Publishing Co., 1927.

Dickey, Marcus. *The Youth of James Whitcomb Riley*. Indianapolis: The Bobbs-Merrill Co., 1919.

Duval, John C. *The Adventures of Big-Foot Wallace, the Texas
Ranger and Hunter*. Edited by Mabel Major and Rebecca
Smith Lee. Lincoln: University of Nebraska Press, 1966.

Francesco, Grete de. *The Power of the Charlatan*. New Haven:
Yale University Press, 1939.

Freeman, Graydon Laverne, *The Medicine Showman*. Watkins
Glen, N.Y.: Century House, 1957.

Gilbert, Douglas. *American Vaudeville*. New York: Dover Publications, Inc., 1963.

Greenwood, Isaac J. *The Circus, Its Origins and Growth Prior to 1835*. New York: The Dunlap Society, 1898.

Harangues, or Speeches, of Several Celebrated Quack-Doctors in Town and Country, The. London, 1762.

Hartt, Rollin Lynde. *The People at Play*. Boston: Houghton Mifflin Co., 1909.

Hechtlinger, Adelaide. *The Great Patent Medicine Era*. New York: Grosset and Dunlap, Inc., 1970.

Holbrook, Stewart H. *The Golden Age of Quackery*. New York: The Macmillan Co., 1959.

Holtman, Jerry. *Freak Show Man*. Los Angeles: Holloway House Publishing Co., 1968.

Hoyt, Harlowe R. *Town Hall Tonight*. New York: Bramhall House, 1955.

Hunt, Charles T., Sr. (as told to John C. Cloutman). *The Story of Mr. Circus*. Rochester, N. H.: The Record Press, 1954.

Hutton, Laurence. *Curiosities of the American Stage*. New York: Harper & Brothers, 1891.

Jameson, Eric. *The Natural History of Quackery*. London: Michael Joseph, 1961.

Kelley, Thomas P., Jr. *The Fabulous Kelley*. Richmond Hill, Ontario: Simon and Schuster of Canada, Ltd., 1968.

Kett, Joseph F. *The Formation of the American Medical Profession*. New Haven: Yale University Press, 1968.

Lewis, Arthur H. *Carnival*. New York: Trident Press, 1970.

Lewis, Sinclair. *Main Street*. New York: Harcourt, Brace & World, Inc., 1920.

McKechnie, Samuel. *Popular Entertainments Through the Ages*. London: Sampson Low, Marston and Co., Ltd., n.d.

McNeal, Violet. *Four White Horses and a Brass Band*. Garden City, N.Y.: Doubleday & Co., Inc., 1947.

Malone, Bill C. *Country Music U.S.A.* Austin: University of Texas Press, 1968.

Miller, John. *A Twentieth Century History of Erie County, Pennsylvania*. Chicago: Lewis Publishing Co., 1909.

Moody, Richard, ed. *Dramas from the American Theatre, 1762–1909*. Cleveland: The World Publishing Company, 1966.

Murray, Keith A. *The Modocs and Their War*. Norman: University of Oklahoma Press, 1959.

Nelson's Biographical Dictionary and Historical Reference Book of Erie County, Pennsylvania. Erie: S. B. Nelson, 1896.

Nevins, Allan. *John D. Rockefeller*. New York: Charles Scribner's Sons, 1941.

Odell, G. C. D. *Annals of the New York Stage.* 15 vols. New York: Columbia University Press, 1927.

O. Henry. [W. S. Porter] *The Gentle Grafter.* New York: Doubleday, Page and Co., 1916.

Oliver, N. T. *Mexican Bill, the Cowboy Detective.* Chicago: Eagle Publishing Co., 1888.

———. *The Priceless Recipes.* Chicago: Laird and Lee, 1900.

Pancoast, Charles L. *Trail Blazers of Advertising.* New York: Frederick H. Hitchcock, 1926.

Pickard, Madge E., and Buley, R. Carlyle. *The Midwest Pioneer, His Ills, Cures, and Doctors.* New York: Henry Schuman, 1946.

Piercy, Harry D. *Shaker Medicine,* reprinted from *Selected Papers,* Shaker Historical Society, October 1957.

Provol, William Lee. *The Pack Peddler.* Greenville, Pa.: The Beaver Printing Company, 1933.

Rose, Will. *The Vanishing Village.* New York: Citadel Press, 1963.

Rourke, Constance. *American Humor.* New York: Harcourt, Brace and Co., Inc., 1931.

Sandberg, Carl. *Always the Young Strangers.* New York: Harcourt, Brace and Co., 1953.

Schaffner, Neil E., with Vance Johnson. *The Fabulous Toby and Me.* Englewood Cliffs, N. J.: Prentice-Hall, Inc., 1968.

Shafer, Henry B. *The American Medical Profession, 1783 to 1850.* New York: Columbia University Press, 1936.

Slout, William Lawrence. *Theatre in a Tent.* Bowling Green, Ohio: Bowling Green University Popular Press, 1972.

Smith, William. *The History of the Province of New-York . . . to the Year M. DCC. XXXII.* London, 1757.

Stone, Fred. *Rolling Stone.* New York: McGraw-Hill Book Co., Inc., 1945.

Taylor, Robert Lewis. *A Journey to Matecumbe.* New York: Avon Books, 1961.

Thompson, C. J. S. *The Quacks of Old London.* London: Brentano's Ltd., 1928.

Wild West, The. Fort Worth: Amon Carter Museum of Western Art, 1970.

Wilson, Harry Leon. *Professor How Could You!* New York: Cosmopolitan Book Corporation, 1924.

Wright, Richardson. *Hawkers and Walkers in Early America.* New York: Frederick Ungar Publishing Co., 1965.

Young, James Harvey. *The Medical Messiahs.* Princeton: Princeton University Press, 1967.

————. *The Toadstool Millionaires.* Princeton: Princeton University Press, 1961.

Zeidman, Irving. *The American Burlesque Show.* New York: Hawthorn Books, Inc., 1967.

Articles

Allen, Ralph. "Our Native Theatre: Honky-Tonk, Minstrel Shows, Burlesque." *The American Theatre: A Sum of Its Parts.* Edited by Henry Williams. New York: Samuel French, Inc., 1971.

Burt, William P. "Back Stage with a Medicine Show Fifty Years Ago." *Colorado Magazine,* July 1942, 127–136.

Cagle, William R. "James Whitcomb Riley: Notes on the Early Years." *Manuscripts,* Spring 1965, 3–11.

Clifford, F. J. "The Medicine Show." *Frontier Times,* December 1930, 92–96.

Cowen, David L. "Colonial Laws Pertaining to Pharmacy." *Journal of the American Pharmaceutical Association,* December 1934, 1236–1242.

Donovan, Richard, and Whitney, Dwight. "Last of America's Tooth Plumbers." *Collier's,* January 5, 12, 19, 1952.

Douglas, W. A. S. "Pitch Doctors." *American Mercury,* February 1927, 222–226.

Edstrom, David. "Medicine Men of the '80's." *Readers Digest,* June 1938, 77–78.

Johnston, Winifred. "Medicine Show." *Southwest Review,* Summer 1936, 390–399.

LeBlanc, Thomas J. "The Medicine Show." *American Mercury,* June 1925, 232–237.

Nathan, George Jean. "The Medicine Man." *Harper's Weekly,* September 9, 1911, p. 24.

Nebel, Long John. "The Pitchman." *Harper's,* May 1961, 50–54.

Nevin, David. "The Brass-Band Pitchman and His Million-Dollar Elixer." *True,* March 1962, 16ff.

Oliver, N. T., as told to Wesley Stout. "Alagazam, The Story of Pitchmen High and Low." *Saturday Evening Post,* October 19, 1929, 26ff.

————., as told to Wesley Stout. "Med Show." *Saturday Evening Post,* September 14, 1929, 12ff.

Petersen, William J. "Patent Medicine Advertising Cards." *The Palimpsest,* June 1969, 317–331.

"Picturesque Medicine Shows Combined Entertainment with Salesmanship." *Missouri Historical Review*, 1951, 374–376.

Reeves, Dorothea D. "Come All for the Cure-all." *Harvard Library
Bulletin*, pp. 253–272.

Sappington, Joe. "The Passing of the Medicine Show." *Frontier
Times*, February 1930, 229–230.

Soucey, Robert. "The Egregious Quacks." *MD*, August 1971, 92–
100.

Taylor, Robert Lewis. "Talker." *The New Yorker*, April 19, 1958,
48ff.

Tully, Jim. "The Giver of Life." *American Mercury*, June 1928.

Young, James Harvey. "American Medical Quackery in the Age
of the Common Man." *Mississippi Valley Historical Review*,
March 1961.

———. "The Hadacol Phenomenon." *Emory University Quarterly*,
June 1951.

———. "The Patent Medicine Almanac." *Wisconsin Magazine of
History*, Spring 1962.

———. "Patent Medicines and Indians." *Emory University Quarterly*,
Summer 1961.

Newspapers

Atlanta *Constitution*, August 19, 1951, and August 24, 1951.

Atlanta *Journal*, August 21, 1951.

Billboard, numbers from 1900 to 1950.

Chicago *Tribune*, July 21, 1931.

Corry *Times-News*, July 9, 1961.

Massachusetts *Spy*, September 5, 1771.

New Haven *Register*, January 16, 1921.

New York *Clipper*, February 24, 1912.

New York *Mercury*, September 17, 1753.

New York *Times*, January 29, 1969.

Patent Medicine Almanacs, Songsters, Books and Magazines

Daring Donald McKay, or the Last War-Trail of the Modocs,
Chicago: Rounds Brothers, 1881.

Eastman, Edwin. *Captured and Branded by the Camanche [sic]
Indians in the Year 1860,* n.p., n.d.

*Enquire Within for Many Useful Facts Relating to Your Health
and Happiness.* New Haven: The Kickapoo Indians, n.d.

First Time of Everything. New Haven: Kickapoo Indian Medicine Co., n.d.

Hamlin's Wizard Oil, the Book of Songs. Chicago: Hamlin's Wizard Oil Co., n.d.

Indian Scout Life. Oregon Indian Medicine Co., n.d.

Kickapoo Indian Dream Book. New Haven: Kickapoo Indian Medicine Co., n.d.

Kickapoo Indian Life and Scenes, n.p., n.d.

Kickapoo Indians and Their Medicine Men, The. New York: Great American Engraving and Printing Co., n.d.

Kickapoo Indians: Life and Scenes Among the Indians. New Haven: Kickapoo Indian Medicine Co., n.d.

Life and Scenes Among the Kickapoo Indians. New Haven: Healy and Bigelow, n.d.

Lighthall, J. I. *The Indian Household Medicine Guide.* Peoria, Ill., 1883.

Solomon, James M., Jr. *Advice to Invalids,* n.p., n.d.

Letters

Barr, Joseph L. Letter to Brooks McNamara, August 26, 1969.

Bartok, Milton. Letter to Brooks McNamara, February 9, 1970.

Clark, Keith. Letter to Brooks McNamara, January 11, 1971.

Cody, William. Letter to William McKay, December 7, no year given.

McKay, Donald. Letters to William McKay, October 24, 1880; April 28, 1888; March 6, 1892.

Noell, Anna Mae. Letters to Brooks McNamara, June 26, 1970; June 15, 1972; July 15, 1972; July 30, 1972; August 12, 1972.

Ruesskamp, William. Letters to Brooks McNamara, May 23, 1970; August 6, 1970.

Sachs, Bill. Letter to Brooks McNamara, June 1, 1970.

Interviews

Bartok, Milton, Mr. and Mrs. Interviewed by Brooks McNamara, April 1970.

Hamilton, Harve. Interviewed by James Harvey Young, 1958.

Lomax, Milton. Interviewed by Brooks McNamara, June 1970.

Mighty Atom. Interviewed by Brooks McNamara, July 1970.

St. John, Flo. Interviewed by Brooks McNamara, April 1970.

Smith, Bill. Interviewed by Brooks McNamara, February 1972.

Snyder, Bobby. Interviewed by Brooks McNamara, April 1970.

Styer, Bob, Mr. and Mrs. Interviewed by Brooks McNamara, July 1970.

Miscellaneous

Gamble, Claude. "The Medicine Show." Manuscript sketch written for the Peoria *Star*. Possession of Robert Gamble, Sea Cliff, New York.

Rinzler, Ralph and Richard, eds. *Notes to Old-Time Music at Clarence Ashley's,* Folkways Records Album FA2355.

Flyers, clippings, showbills, advertising cards, circulars, photographs, blank forms, labels, medicine boxes, etc., in the Helfand Scrapbook and the various collections noted in the Preface.

INDEX